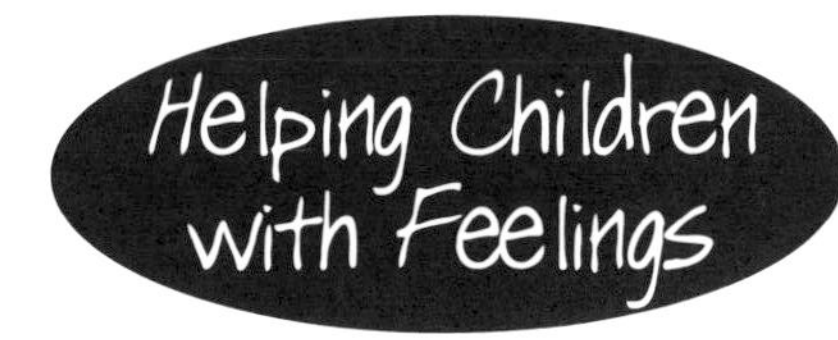

Helping Children who are Anxious or Obsessional

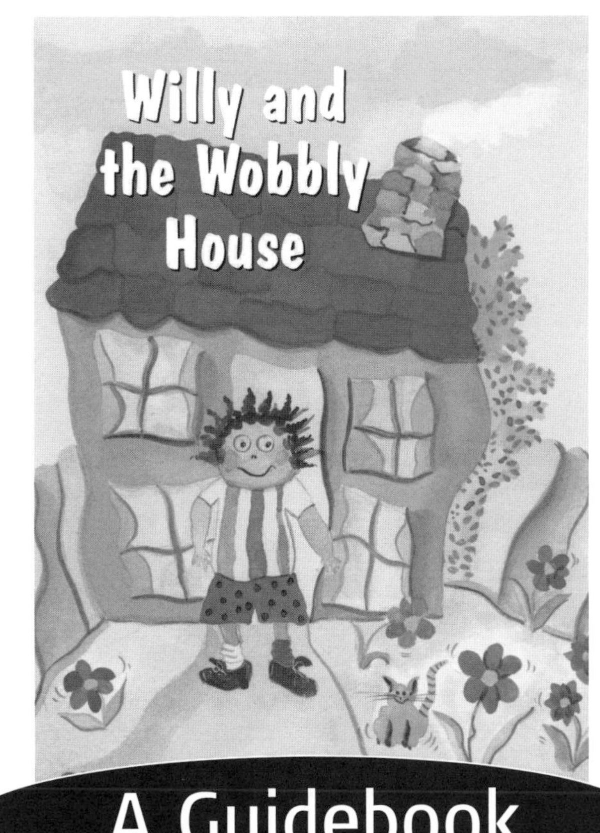

A Guidebook

Margot Sunderland

Illustrated by

Nicky Armstrong

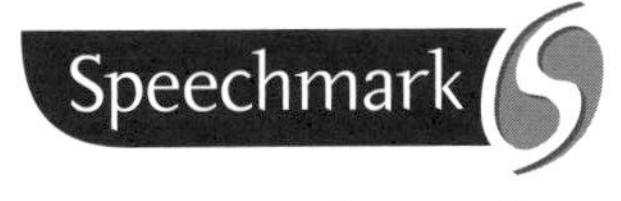

www.speechmark.net

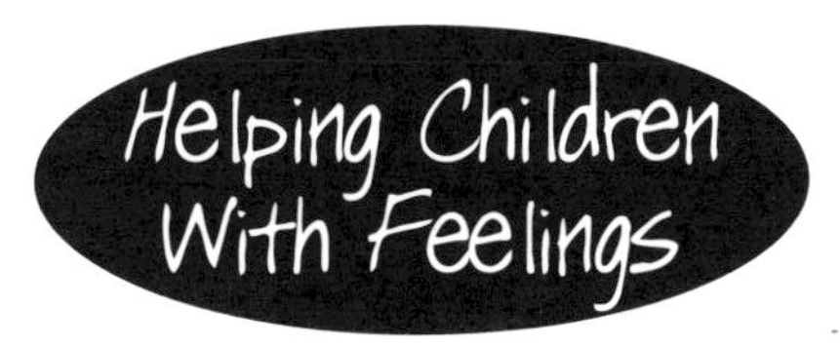

Helping Children who are Anxious or Obsessional

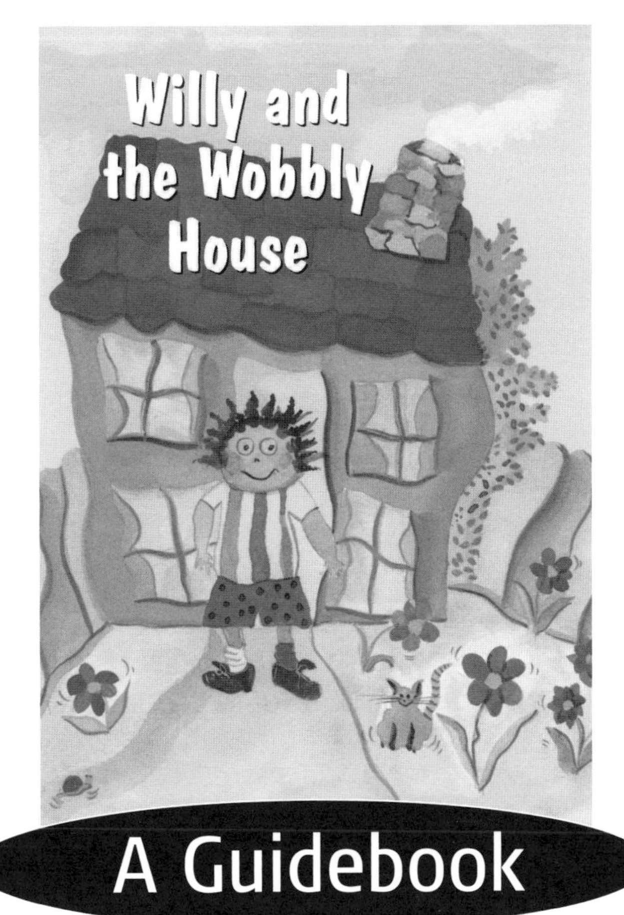

A Guidebook

Dedication

For Paulo

Note on the Text

For the sake of clarity alone, throughout the text the child has been referred to as 'he' and the parent as 'she'.

Unless otherwise stated, for clarity alone, where 'mummy', 'mother' or 'mother figure' is used, this refers to either parent or other primary caretaker.

Confidentiality

Where appropriate, full permission has been granted by adults, or children and their parents, to use clinical material. Other illustrations comprise synthesised and disguised examples to ensure anonymity.

Published by
Speechmark Publishing Ltd
Sunningdale House, 43 Caldecotte Lake Drive, Milton Keynes MK7 8LF, United Kingdom
Tel: +44 (0)1908 277177 Fax: +44 (0)1908 278297
www.speechmark.net

First published 2000
Reprinted 2002, 2004, 2005, 2007, 2008, 2009, 2011, 2012

002-5059/Printed in the United Kingdom by Hobbs

British Library Cataloguing in Publication Data
Sunderland, Margot
Willy and the wobbly house : helping children who are anxious or obsessional Guidebook. – (Stories for Troubled Children)
1. Storytelling – Therapeutic use 2. Child psychology
3. Learning, Psychology of
I. Title II. Armstrong, Nicky
615.8'516

ISBN 978 0 86388 454 2

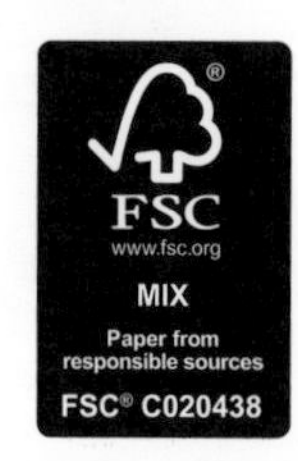

Contents

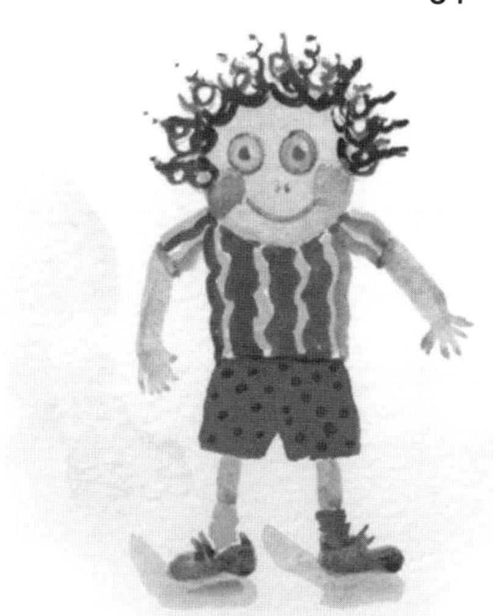

ABOUT THE AUTHOR

MARGOT SUNDERLAND is Founding Director of the Centre for Child Mental Health, London. She is also Head of the Children and Young People Section of The United Kingdom Association for Therapeutic Counselling. In addition, she formed the research project, 'Helping Where it Hurts' which offers free therapy and counselling to troubled children in several primary schools in North London. She is a registered Integrative Arts Psychotherapist and registered Child Therapeutic Counsellor, Supervisor and Trainer.

Margot is also Principal of The Institute for Arts in Therapy and Education – a fully accredited Higher Education College running a Diploma course in Child Therapy and Masters Degree courses in Arts Psychotherapy and Arts in Education and Therapy.

Margot is a published poet and author of two non-fiction books – one on *Dance* (Routledge Theatre Arts, New York and J Garnet Miller, England) and the other called *Draw on Your Emotions* (Speechmark Publishing, Milton Keynes and Erickson, Italy).

ABOUT THE ILLUSTRATOR

NICKY ARMSTRONG holds an MA from The Slade School of Fine Art and a BA Hons in Theatre Design from the University of Central England. She is currently teacher of trompe l'œil at The Hampstead School of Decorative Arts, London. She has achieved major commissions nationally and internationally in mural work and fine art.

ACKNOWLEDGEMENTS

A special acknowledgement to Mattan Lederman who, at age seven, drew an entire set of pictures for all of the five stories in the pack. Several of his ideas and designs were then adopted by the illustrator.

I would like to thank Katherine Pierpont, Charlotte Emmett and Ruth Bonner for all their superb skill and rigour in the editing process, and for making the long writing journey such a pleasurable one.

I would also like to thank all the children, trainees and supervisees with whom I have worked, whose poetry, images and courage have greatly enriched both my work and my life.

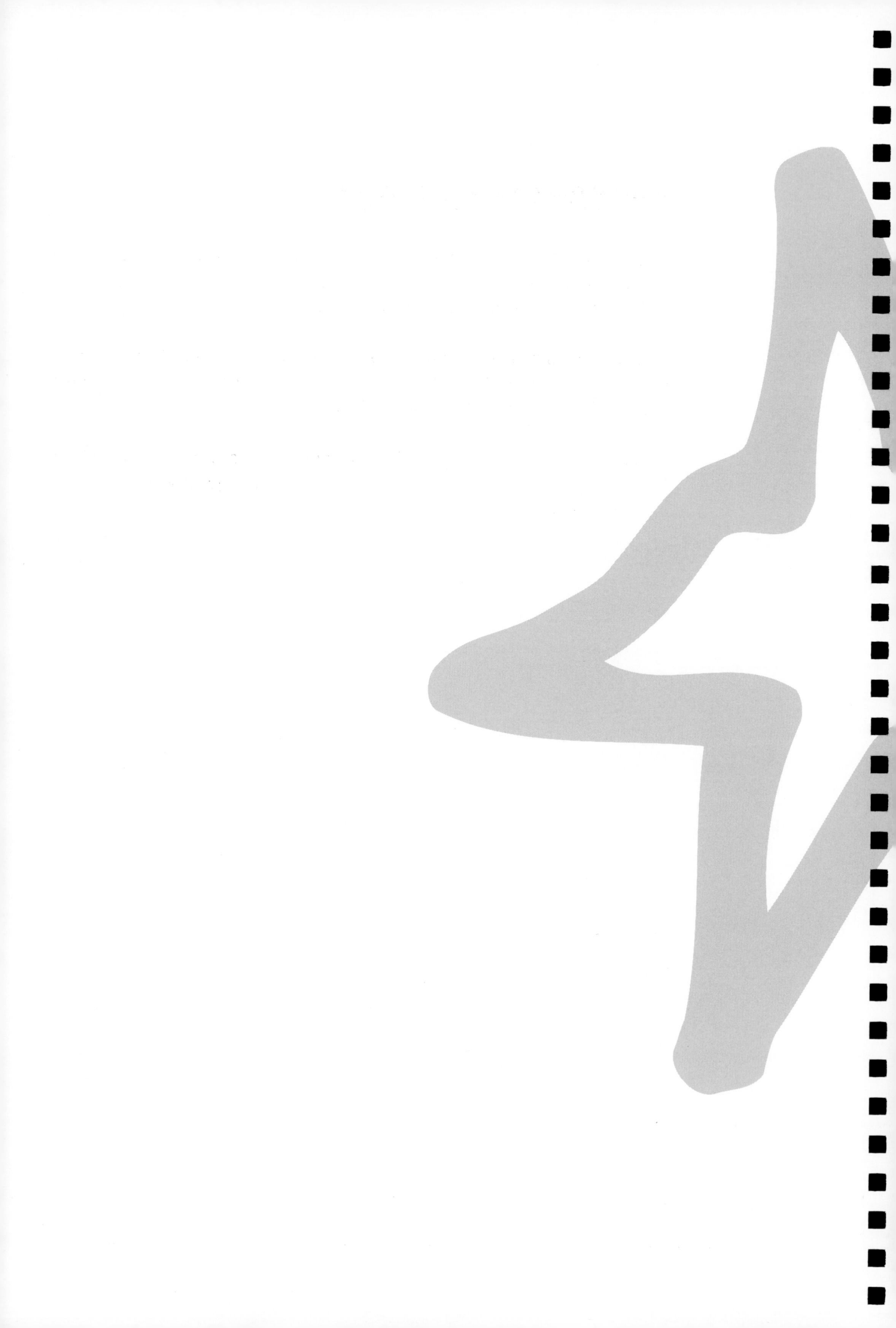

ABOUT THIS GUIDEBOOK

If a child is going to benefit from the full therapeutic potential of *Willy and the Wobbly House*, this accompanying guidebook will be a vital resource. We strongly advise that you read it before reading the story itself to the child. By doing so, you will come to the child from a far more informed position, and so you will be able to offer him a far richer, and more empathic, response.

This guidebook details the common psychological origins and most relevant psychotherapeutic theories for the problems and issues addressed in the story. If you read it before reading the story to the child, it will prevent your coming to the child from an ignorant or closed viewpoint about why he is troubled. For example, 'I'm sure that Johnny's school work has gone downhill because he is missing his Daddy, who moved out a few months ago', may be an accurate or inaccurate hypothesis. There may be many other reasons for Johnny's problems with his school work, which have not been considered. The problem may well be complex, as are so many psychological problems. Coming from a closed or too narrow viewpoint all too often means that the helping adult is in danger of projecting on to the child *their own* feelings and views of the world.

Very few parents are consciously cruel. When something goes wrong in the parenting of a child, it is often to do with the parent *not knowing* about some vital aspect of child psychology or child development, or a lack in the way the parent was brought up themselves. There is still a tragic gap between what is known about effective parenting in child psychology, psychotherapy and scientific research, and how much of this is communicated to parents via parenting books, or through television and the press. So this guidebook is not about blaming parents. Rather, the aim is to support them. More generally, the aim is to heighten the awareness of *anyone* looking after children about how things can go wrong (usually despite the best intentions), and about how to help them go right in the first place, or to get mended if they do go wrong.

This guidebook includes what children themselves have said about what it is like for them coping with the problems and issues addressed in the story, and describes the stories children have enacted through their play. It also includes a section that offers you suggestions and ideas for things to say and things to do after you have read *Willy and the Wobbly House* to the child. The suggestions and ideas are specifically designed to help a child to think about, express and further digest his feelings about the problems and issues addressed in the story. Some of the ideas and exercises are also designed to inspire children to speak more about what they are feeling through *their own* spontaneous story-making.

Everyday language is not the natural language for children to use to speak about what they feel. But, with an adult they trust, they can usually show or enact, draw or play out their feelings very well indeed. Therefore, many of the exercises offered in this guidebook will support the child in creative, imaginative and playful ways of expressing himself. Also, so that you avoid asking too many questions, interrogating the child about his feeling life (to which children do not respond at all well) some of the exercises simply require the child to tick a box, 'show me' or pick a word or an image from a selection.

INTRODUCTION

What the story is about

Willy is an anxious little boy who experiences the world as a very unsafe and wobbly place, where something bad might happen at any minute. Joe, the boy next door, is too ordered and tidy to be able to relax and really enjoy life. Willy longs for order. Joe longs for things to wobble. They both think that their own experience is just the way life is, so they had better get used to it.

But when they meet Mrs Flop from the post office, she tells them that they do not have to put up with feeling as they do, and that they should visit the Puddle People who live behind the big red bin in the park. With new hope, Willy and Joe go off together to find the bin. They meet the Puddle People, who help them to break out of their fixed patterns, and find far richer ways of being in the world.

The main psychological messages in this story

If being yourself is a wobbly matter, then being in the world becomes a wobbly business too.

If being yourself is a too tight, boring or narrow affair, then being in the world can feel like that too.

With help, it is possible to break out of a 'little life' into an expansive way of being in the world.

Your main way of being is not the only one available to you. It is not true that you are stuck with an experience of self that you do not like. Change is possible.

If you can find them, certain relationship experiences can expand your way of being, beyond your wildest dreams.

It is all too easy to get stuck in a certain way of being, and then think that this is all there is.

Who the story is for

This story was written for children like Willy:

Children who are insecure.

Children who feel too wobbly inside.

Children who feel anxious a lot of the time.

Children who worry too much.

Children who suffer from phobias or nightmares.

Children who do not know calmness.

Children who find it difficult to concentrate.

Children who are wobbly because they live in an upside-down world.

Children who have suffered a trauma.

and for children like Joe:

Children who feel dull.

Children who are worryingly good.

Children who feel too ordered or tidied up inside.

Children who live in their heads.

Children who use order and routine as a way of coping with 'messy' feelings.

Children who retreat into dullness as a way of managing their being in the world.

Children who fear feeling too much life.

Children who develop obsessive–compulsive behaviour in order to ward off their too-powerful feelings.

Children who seem like little adults.

Children who find it difficult to let go and have fun.

First we will look at understanding and working with children like Willy, and then we will look at understanding and working with children like Joe.

UNDERSTANDING WHAT LIFE IS LIKE FOR CHILDREN WHO FEEL TOO WOBBLY INSIDE

> Her life was turning, turning,
> In mazes of heat and sound.
> But for peace her soul was yearning.
> (Matthew Arnold, 'Requiescat', cited in Quiller-Couch, 1979)

Feeling wobbly inside can show itself in children through a variety of anxious symptoms, such as phobias, psychosomatic symptoms, obsessive-compulsive rituals, bed-wetting and nightmares. Wobbly children can find it difficult to concentrate. They can seem agitated a lot of the time because they are so unsettled inside. Wobbly feelings all too easily snatch the child's attention away from his outer world, as there is too much going on in his inner world. Some feel too anxious to explore the world or to be at all adventurous, and so cling to a parent or to home – the known, the familiar. Other wobbly children may lash out because they feel too wobbly inside and are unable to manage the intensity of their feelings:

> I was overwhelmed by chaotic feelings, which I discharged in an orgy of smashing. (Little, 1990, p100)

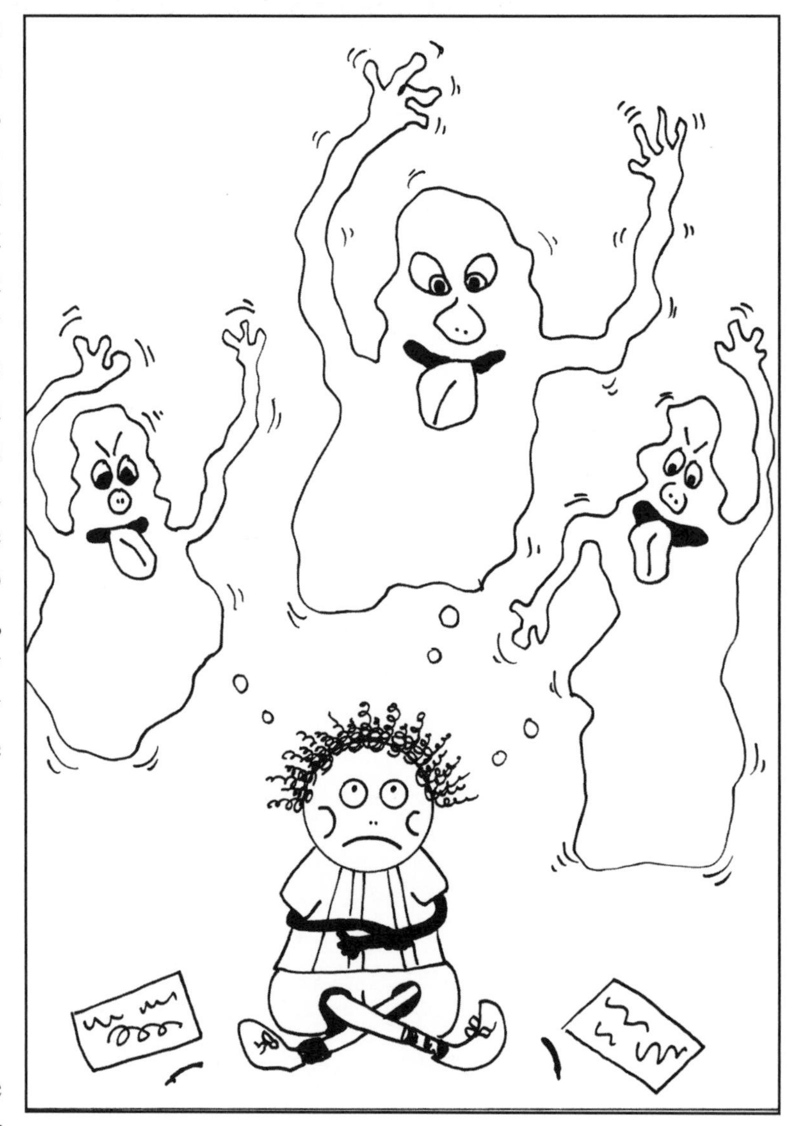

Figure 1 All about Willy

Some children feel wobbly because they do not know who they are. Their sense of self is very fragile. One ten-year-old boy called Tomas said, 'There is no one "me". It makes everything feel very upside-downy.' He complained of there being too little sense of continuity of himself over time 'I never feel I'm quite the Tomas I was yesterday or last week.' Such children can feel all over the place, particularly in stressful situations as there is no central, organising self to be stable. When a child does not know who he is, he often does not know what he feels either. This also makes him vulnerable to feeling the feelings of the people around him. For example, Polly, aged twelve, had no stable sense of who she was, no central organising core self. So each time she watched television she would present herself for a while afterwards like someone from the television programme. After a cowboy movie she would be aggressive, after a love story tender, after a comedy programme, light and jovial. Of course, it is a very wobbly thing to not know who you are or what you feel. Some children who are wobbly are very untidy. Their inner muddle of wobbly feelings needs an echo in their outer life. They feel at home in mess. It is a mirror of what they are feeling inside. Some children who are wobbly suffer from a mind clutter of ruminations, circular thoughts or different 'voices' running round their heads. This is known as 'mind noise'. Mind noise can feel like interference on the radio, cluttering clear perception of feelings and thoughts. It is very tiring and drains concentration.

Some people find it very difficult being with an anxious, wobbly child, because they end up feeling all the child's wobbliness too. The energy of the child's anxiety enters the atmosphere too powerfully. So wobbly children can end up feeling avoided rather than helped. Some people, as Segal says, 'feel so messed up inside that they seem to have to make everyone around them feel messed up too' (1985, p77). Children living with too much wobbliness, too much anxiety, can believe that 'No one will be able to cope with the mess that is me, so I'd better just manage it all by myself.' This is sometimes a projection. Because the child himself cannot manage the mess of his too many, too strong feelings, and the mess in his mind, he assumes that others cannot either.

Worry as a particularly wobbly feeling

> One day [Mr Worry] went for a walk. He was worried that he might walk too far and not be able to get home, but on the other hand, he was worried that if he didn't walk far enough, he wouldn't get enough exercise. He hurried along, worrying. Or you could say, he worried along hurrying. (Hargreaves, 1978, p11)

Many children who feel wobbly inside find the world a very worrying place. Some wobbly children worry about everything: they worry about home, they worry about school; they worry about friends going off them, they worry about being ill or dying. In short, such children are not at peace.

Some wobbly children are full of worry about their sense of worth: 'Does my Mummy love me?'; 'Will my Mummy leave me?'; 'Will my Mummy stop loving me if I fail my exams?' Other wobbly children have worrying thoughts such as, 'Are Mummy and Daddy going to split up?' or 'Is Mummy going to die?' One little boy, whose Daddy had had heartburn one night, spent a lot of time at school in his craft lesson the next day trying to mend 'the heart' that he had made. But it kept breaking. The teacher said it was desperate to watch.

Other children worry about a 'broken Mummy' because their Mummy has been ill or suffered an accident. One little girl whose Mummy had lost her two front teeth in a fight kept drawing mouths and teeth for weeks afterwards, until a counsellor helped her work through her grief and worry about what it felt like to have a broken Mummy.

Anxiety and worry are often defences against fear, terror or nameless dread. Freud realised this in 1923 when he said, 'anxiety protects us from our fear'. Anxiety can also be a defence against other too strong feelings, such as love, hate, rage or desire. Strong feelings such as these are experienced as dangerous by the child because of their sheer intensity, as we will examine later.

> My thoughts were like unbridled children, grown
> Too headstrong for their mother.
> (Shakespeare, *Troilus and Cressida*, III, 2, vv119–20)

Understanding why children like Willy feel so wobbly

Children can be wobbly because they have not found something calm or soothing enough in the adults in their lives

Without sufficient soothing and calm, babies can develop very anxious wobbly selves. This is because babies are born extremely hypersensitive. They are very fragile psychologically as well as physically. The baby's self is not yet integrated. Research shows that a week after birth, when the soothing chemicals of birth (endorphins) have worn off, a baby's stress hormones (cortisol) are way above the norm. They are in an acutely stressed state. It is as if they are saying 'Help! Help!'

As Freud says, a baby comes into the world 'not quite finished'. As well as his body, his brain and central nervous system are still developing. For the first few weeks, a baby's vision is very blurred, too. All in all, the baby is an unintegrated self and can 'fall apart' very easily. Think of a young baby having its nappy changed; being put into the bath or being undressed. The desperate howling is often due to a parent not realising just how acutely sensitive babies are; how all acts such as these must be carried out with exquisite sensitivity, slowness and calmness. Otherwise the baby simply moves into a state of fragmentation. Furthermore, a baby's world is one of feelings, sensations and energies. He cannot yet make sense of and order his experiences through thinking. And so his intense feeling states often threaten to overwhelm him. He *must* get help with these. He simply cannot manage them on his own. All babies are 'on fire' at times, from the sheer intensity of their need, rage, frustration and desperation. At these times babies need to meet with a stilling 'water', gently lapping, gently holding, in the form of a very soothing parent.

Still

I am this blizzard of rush for you,
Hurtling spill of love and squall
Right over you, all over you.
And you there
Still there.
This pool of you,
This pool of still.
As if to take me there
As if to take me there.

Margot Sunderland

Some people say, 'Let your baby cry himself to sleep'; 'You'll spoil him if you pick him up all the time. He'll never be able to separate from you if you pick him up immediately every time he cries'; 'If you let him sleep in your bed, you'll get a clingy child. You're making a rod for your own back', or 'The baby is only trying to control you by crying.' The facts are as follows. The foetus knows nothing of a non-enveloping world. Rather, the foetus is part of his mother. He is merged with her, in a state of 'inter-penetrating mix up', as the psychoanalyst Michael Balint (1955) calls it. Fortunate babies are born into a world *not unlike that of the womb*, where they feel enveloped by the warm skin of their mother's body, where they feel emotionally 'held' in both her heart and her mind, without feeling that they fall out of either, metaphorically speaking.

Many unfortunate babies, whose parents do not fully realise the necessity of this vital continuity between the world of the womb and the outside world, move from the warmth, the holding and the safety of the womb to times of terrifying isolation, of feeling held by nothing, attached to nothing. When a baby is left too long on his own without being held, touched or comforted, you can hear from the intensity of his cries how desperate he is to recover the warm, safe world of direct closeness with the soothing calmness of another's body. This crying is often the sound of – massive alarm, of urgent protest – a survival cry. A baby's cry *is* as bad as it sounds. Babies have no concept of time, so a parent's leaving for a few minutes can feel utterly terrifying, as if she has gone forever. For example, a baby may be with his mother having an intimate time, when she suddenly has to leave to answer the door-bell. The baby cannot make the connection between a bell ringing and his mother disappearing, he just knows that his mother has disappeared and that she may well have gone forever. As Freud says, the baby 'cannot as yet distinguish between temporary absence and permanent loss. As soon as it loses sight of its mother it behaves as if it were never going to see her again' (1926 [1979, p330]).

So what happens if the baby is not only full of his own too-intense feeling states, but those of his mother are also too strong, too jarring, or too harsh? If this is the case, he lives in a very frightening world, because, in many senses, the baby, like the foetus, is still part of his mother's body. The baby is acutely sensitive to his mother's emotional energies, qualities of feeling, the intensities and urgencies of her movements, her 'atmospheres'. Daniel Stern, a famous infant-mother researcher, calls the energetic states and movement qualities to which the baby is so acutely sensitive, 'vitality affects':

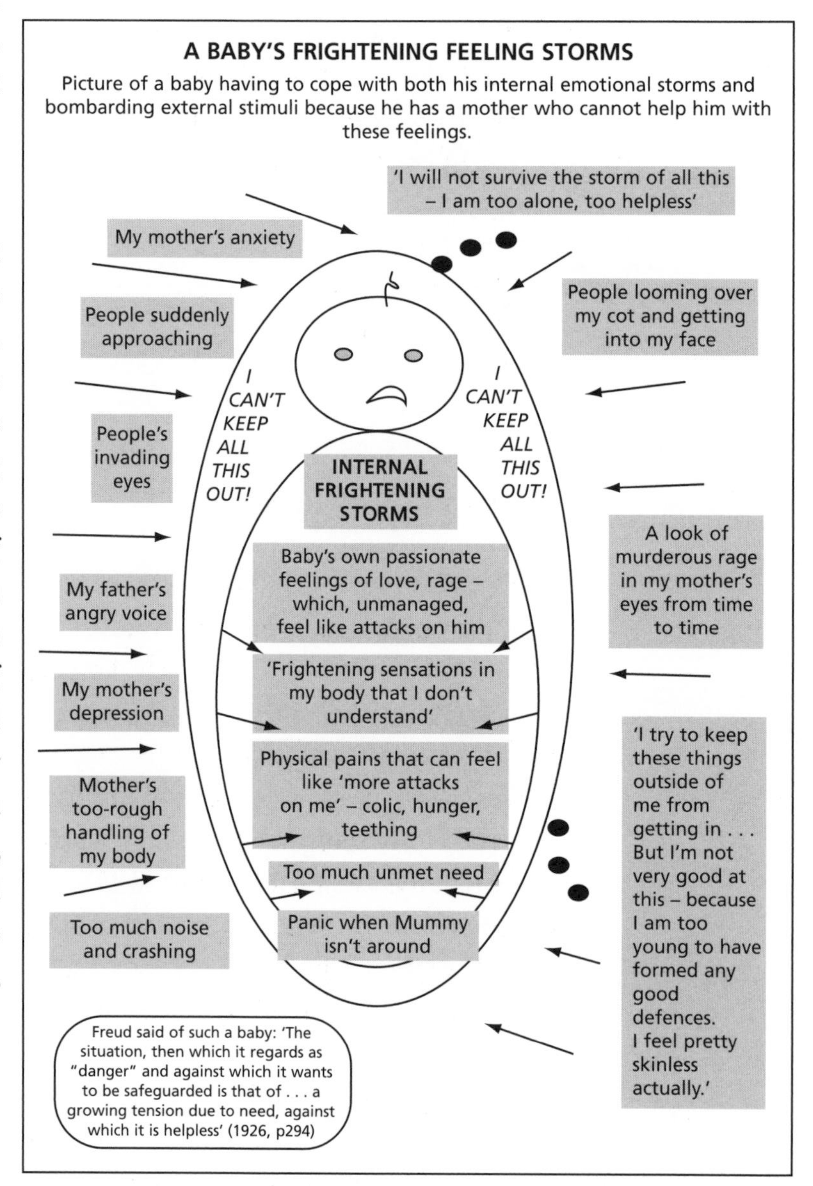

Figure 2 A baby's frightening feeling storms

> These elusive qualities are better captured by terms such as 'surging', 'fading away', 'fleeting', 'explosive', 'crescendo', 'decrescendo', 'bursting', 'drawn out'. The infant experiences these qualities from within, as well as in the behaviour of other persons. Different feelings of vitality can be expressed in a multitude of parental acts – how the mother picks up the baby, folds the diapers, grooms her hair or the baby's hair, reaches for the bottle, unbuttons her blouse. The infant is immersed in these feelings. (Stern, 1985, p54)

If his mother's energies are calm energies, they can become his calm energies. He can feel deeply soothed by them, sometimes even reach intense states of bliss or peace. Her energies can calm him out of his most unmanageable states of inner tension. If, however, her energies are not calm, but rather anxious, chaotic or fraught, he can feel extremely disturbed by them. He can feel all her jarring emotional energies in his little body-mind (as yet with no defences), and often at a far higher volume and intensity than she herself does. At times, he may feel consumed by her harsh intensities, overtaken by them. Think of swimming in the sea. In one sense you are in a merged state with the water. You are part of it. Then imagine the huge force of a coming wave that sends you right under the water. It is a bit like that. (See Figures 2 and 3.)

A BABY WHO HAS A MOTHER TO HELP HIM WITH HIS EXTERNAL FEELING STORMS AND EXTERNAL FEELING STORMS
'Mummy protects me by making sure she doesn't put any of her own anxious, frightened or angry feelings on to me, so I don't have to deal with them as well as my own.'
'I find ways to let my mother know about the frightening feeling storms inside me, and get her to help me with them so I can get on with developing a strong sense of self, instead of having to fend off frightening feelings inside me and outside of me.'
A CALM SOOTHING MOTHER
'Mummy protects me from all things too jarring, too harsh, too intrusive, too loud in my outer world. She is very careful how she picks me up, how she speaks to me and how she looks at me. She realises that I am very fragile psychologically as well as physically.'

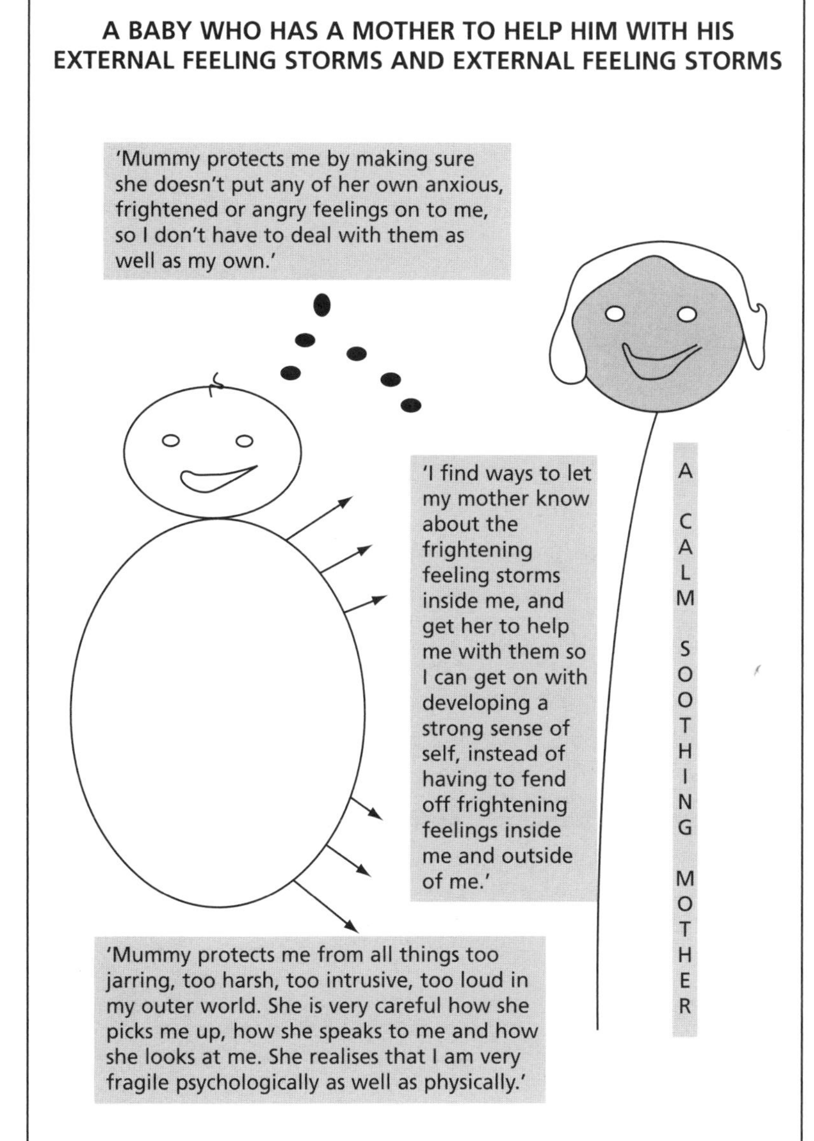

Figure 3 A baby who has a mother to help him with his internal feeling storms and external stimulus storms

If a baby is not to grow up wobbly, he needs a very harmonious environment, not dissimilar to the calm, liquid world of the womb. He needs the change-over from womb to world to be exquisitely gentle, from being a merged water-creature (in the womb), to being a separate creature on dry land: no shocks, no suddenness, no jarring intensities in his mother or other adult, nothing to feel like 'hard edges'.

Similarly, if children are not to grow up wobbly and anxious, they need repeated experience of being comforted by someone who is both strong enough (psychologically speaking) and calm enough. They need to merge their anxious minds and bodies with the calmness and stillness of that adult, until it becomes *their* calmness, *their* stillness. They need to be on the receiving end of the blissful experience of drinking in soothing from an adult who is sufficiently at peace with herself to be able to repeatedly offer them this.

> Their self-confidence as they carried us when we were babies, their security when they allowed us to merge our anxious selves with their tranquillity – via calm voices or via our closeness with their relaxed bodies as they held us – will be retained by us as the calmness we experience as we live our lives. (Kohut & Wolf, 1978, p417)

A child cannot find a natural calmness in himself, or a real sense of inner peace, if he has never known deep calm in his mother; if he has never felt 'gathered in', emotionally speaking, by a mother who could soothe and hold and calm him, if he has too rarely merged himself, felt himself part of *her* strength and *her* calm. In fact, consistently repeated experiences of a soothing adult can leave such a powerful impression on a child that a deep and enduring sense of security ensues. This can have a lifelong effect on the chemical balance in his brain. There is much neurobiological evidence for this (see Schore, 1994; Siegel, 1999; Panksepp, 1998).

Sometimes 'wobbly children' who have not felt 'held together' by a parent in this way gravitate to an object or ritual that will 'hold them together'. For example, one very wobbly, anxious little boy called Robert said that he only felt OK at school if he could sit in the same seat every day, directly by the door and hold on to the blackboard eraser.

> A baby will focus on some continuous sensory stimulus, like a light or a noise, as a way of clinging when not being held by mother. For Ben, in the first few months of his life, I felt the stillness of the object was also important, like someone in a storm-tossed boat trying to focus his eyes on the horizon. (Glucksman, 1987, p348)

The following is an example of a very wobbly boy who failed to receive sufficient soothing from his home environment, but who did receive it from someone at his school:

George, aged six

George, a very anxious and wobbly boy, diagnosed as having Attention Deficit Hyperactivity Disorder (ADHD), would rush from classroom to classroom, throw himself on the floor and say 'Boo! It's me!' Of course, this disrupted people's teaching. He was punished. So, for a long time, he had no one to read his communications; no one said, 'I wonder what you are trying to tell us.' His mother was depressed. He could never gain her attention, except by being naughty.

Luckily, one day George met a school help – a lovely, soothing woman called Betty. When Betty saw George getting more and more agitated, she would pick him up and put him on her knee. George started to go to Betty every day for cuddles, or when he was upset. The manic behaviour stopped when George's desperate call of 'See me! See me!' was heard. George felt very seen by Betty, and very soothed.

Children who are wobbly because their parents are wobbly

If a child has had too many fraught interactions with a too anxious parent figure, or one who has unpredictable energetic shifts, he may well build up a picture of the world (at least in part) as an anxiety-provoking place, and of life as a basically unsafe affair. (This is particularly so in the absence of any other calming, central parent figure, to compensate for, or dilute, these fraught interactions.) In other words, he will build up a picture of the world as being like his anxious parent – a place where nothing is stable or still or constant; a place where anything could happen at any time; a place where everything, metaphorically speaking, is built on sand, or bits of broken glass; a place where he must be on guard.

When children have very anxious parents, their perception of the world is also likely to have been highly coloured by having taken on doom-laden parental messages (verbal or non-verbal) about the world being a scary or dangerous place. Below are common 'frightened' beliefs, which neurotically anxious parents often convey to their children in one form or another:

> If you do something wrong, or make a mistake, it's awful, so try to be perfect.
>
> Don't relax, because that's just when things go wrong.

Be safe, not sorry.

Taking risks will only lead to something bad.

It is a terrible thing not to have security/money/a partner/a home/a job, so stick to them like glue.

In fact, research shows that children often have the very same fears or phobias as their parents – and sometimes in a more extreme form.

> In a study of 70 pre-school children, aged from two to six years, and their mothers, Hagman (1932) found significant correlation between the children who feared dogs and the mothers who feared dogs, and also between children and mothers who feared insects. A correlation was also present, though of lower degree, between children and mothers who feared thunderstorms. (Bowlby, 1973, p160)

One main focus for a parent's neurotic anxiety can be the child himself. (We are talking here of intense and preoccupying anxiety states, rather than common and very natural parental fears.) A common preoccupying fear is that her child will die, or get injured in some awful way. For some children, the effect of being such a central focus for a parent's fear (even when this is unspoken) can be to see the world as a very frightening, unsafe place, where something awful could happen at any moment. This is described very eloquently by Balint: 'Instead of live infants, they were seen, perhaps, as frightening objects who might easily die, and so [these children] experienced their mothers and the world in which they were living as full of dread and fear' (1993, p108).

If a child feels wobbly around his parent, he can feel wobbly around everything. Mummy or Daddy, or both, are the child's secure base for being in the world. So when Mummy or Daddy are *not* a secure base, but are themselves wobbly, then everything in the world can seem wobbly.

Terry, aged seven

Terry is a very anxious child. One day his Mummy is a loving, emotionally present Mummy, the next she is totally preoccupied with her worries and fears and pays him very little attention. So for a day or so Terry has a soft, kind Mummy and then, for the next, he has a rather cold, distant one. Her mood is so changeable that Terry experiences the world as very changeable too. There is something too wobbly, too precarious in his Mummy's love for him. He feels he might lose it any minute. His Mummy complains that Terry is far too clingy: why doesn't he just grow up?

The problem is that if a parent is full of her own anxiety she will not have the mind-space to help her child with his anxiety, so he is left alone with it. As Freud says, 'The child is really not equipped to master psychically the large sums of excitation that reach him whether from without or from within' (1926 [1979, p305]). So without her help, in the form of calm and soothing, he is left battling on his own with his often too intense, too unmanageable feelings. Anxiety is a symptom resulting from this. Furthermore, an anxious or emotionally needy parent can place huge demands (spoken or unspoken) upon her child. This is because such a child can learn how to soothe his anxious mother for *his own* emotional protection. So his own feelings must be pushed even more underground. This never works. Pushed down feelings leak out in all manner of neurotic and/or physical symptoms.

Sally, aged six

Sally's parents were very anxious people. Sally found school a far too anxiety-making affair, and often felt confused or overwhelmed. One day at school, Sally's teacher said, 'Draw something about your life.' Sally did a 'tea' drawing (see Figure 4). The teacher thought the drawing was silly. It was, in fact, a profoundly perceptive statement for this six year-old. Sally could not have described more succinctly the very essence of her life experience at the time. Her 'tea' picture describes a particular time each day when she did not feel anxious, wobbly or overwhelmed. At the end of the day, her father would say, 'Let's all have a cup of tea.' Teatime felt like a safe, clear place: known, regular, real and secure. But surrounding the 'oasis of tea' in her picture was a scribble. The scribble is the overwhelming confusion she felt, living in a family that, while very well-meaning, did not have the resources to her help with her feelings and emotional needs.

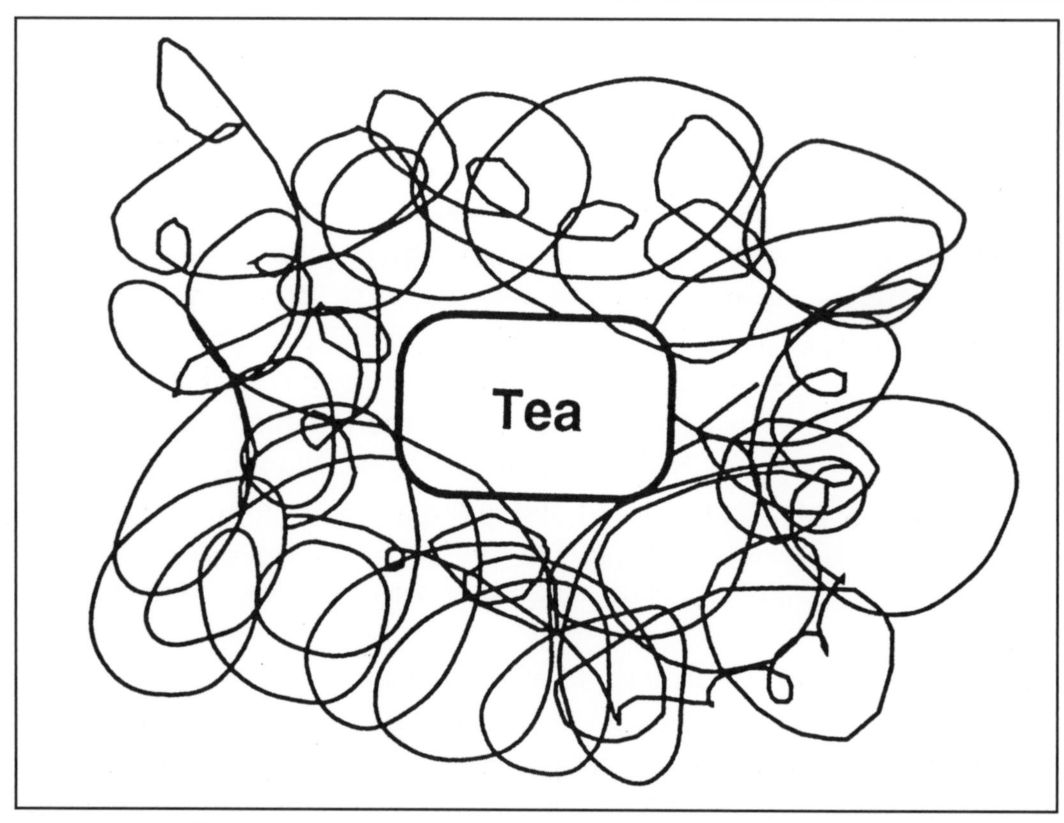

Figure 4 Sally's tea drawing

> Each individual has in all probability a limit beyond which his mental apparatus fails in its function of mastering the quantities of excitation which require to be disposed of. (Freud, 1926 [1979, p305])

To summarise, the parental behaviours that are likely to result in a child feeling wobbly inside:

Over anxious	Unpredictable	Angry
Needy	Demanding	Clingy to him
Over attentive	Emotionally fragile	Frightening
Agitated	Depressed	
Shaming	Emotionally absent	

Furthermore:

> The anxious child may well have too many painful or difficult interactions with a parent-figure who is too full of their own unprocessed feelings, such as anxiety, anger or depression. So the child ends up having to cope with his parent's intense, raw (and often infantile) feelings, as well as trying to manage his own! Consequently, he has had to hold himself together in the face of a 'Mummy-world' or a 'Daddy-world' that he has experienced as just too threatening, confused and/or fragile.

If these painful, difficult interactions happen at a time when the child is still forming vital neuronal connections in his brain for emotional regulation (age 0 to 3, see Schore, 1994), they can have a powerful effect on him psychobiochemically. If too much stress hormone (cortisol) is released during this time, and not enough natural opiates, he can grow up anxious and agitated.

Some children are wobbly because they are not sure whether their Mummy loves them or not: 'Love makes the world a safer place. It means we do not have to hide. It means we can come out to play with all the people everywhere, at home, on earth and in ourselves' (Herman, 1988, p146).

In contrast we now provide a summary of the kind of parenting that is likely to make a child feel secure and safe:

'All of us, from the cradle to the grave, are happiest when life is organised as a series of excursions, long or short, from the secure base provided by our attachment figures' (Bowlby, 1988, p62).

The secure child has been able to 'love in peace'. He has not been frightened of his parents, or made anxious by their anxiety or fragility. He is not worried that either of them might suddenly stop loving him, or that they will love him only conditionally. So in adulthood, he can also 'love in peace'.

The secure child has experienced a parent who has been able consistently to reflect on his emotional states. She has had the mental and emotional space to do this because she is not full of her own unprocessed feelings, or when she is, she gets someone to help her process them. The secure child turns to his parent for soothing and help when he is frightened or upset, because he knows that his parent will be responsive.

The secure child grows up to feel 'bold in his explorations of the world' (Bowlby, 1988, p124). This is because he has the capacity to keep a warm, loving mother in mind when she is not present. This capacity starts to become really firm from around the age of three-and-a-half, when the child can manage from half to whole days away from his most important attachment figures without separation anxiety.

These early, potently good interactions with his parent influence the child's world view so powerfully that, if he is in actual danger (for example in a country at war), he is likely to feel safe because he is with his loving, soothing parent. In contrast, wobbly, insecure children who are in no *actual* danger can feel very unsafe, because they have had no experience of a parent as a secure base, as their very foundation for being in the world. Without the firm foundations laid down by a secure attachment in childhood as described here, there will always be neurotic anxiety. However, children who have not had this foundation in security can be given a second chance through therapy or counselling.

The secure child grows up to see the world as a place with enough hope and goodness to ensure that, with the support of others, even the most awful situations can be endured. As Klein says, 'If love has not been smothered under resentment, grievances and hatred, but has been firmly established in the mind, trust in other people and belief in one's own goodness are like a rock which withstands the blows of circumstance' (1932, p341).

The secure child grows up to see the world as a place where he does not have to 'go it alone' – where there will always be someone he can go to for soothing, help and understanding.

> So deeply established are his expectations and so repeatedly have they been confirmed that, as an adult, he finds it difficult to imagine any other kind of world. This gives him an almost unconscious assurance that, whenever and wherever he might be in difficulty, there are always trustworthy figures available who will come to his aid. He will therefore approach the world with confidence and when faced with potentially alarming situations, is likely to tackle them effectively or to seek help in doing so. (Bowlby, 1973, p208)

How a child senses his parent's unexpressed, brushed-under-the-carpet fears and anxieties

Young children are very open and undefended, and hence easily affected by their parent's emotional energies and mood states. If the parent's inner world is full of too much unprocessed fear or anxiety, then the child's outer world can feel frightening and anxious. Children can often sense their parents' worries, problems and fears. Although these may never be overtly spoken about, the child picks them up acutely at a subliminal level. Looked at another way, there is commonly an 'underground' communication from the parent's unconscious to the child's unconscious. Because of the closeness of many parent-child relationships, this communication is often quite dramatic. As a result, a child can easily end up feeling burdened by the unexpressed anxieties or denied fears of his parent, as well as those that are being overtly expressed. This burden can remain with the child right into his adulthood, coming out as free-floating anxiety ready to attach itself to anything in its path.

Clara, aged four

Clara was referred for therapy because she was very wobbly indeed. She could not concentrate on her schoolwork, clung to teachers and was very agitated. She had a bereaved and deeply grieving mother who had too few people in her life to whom she could take her feelings. Eventually, the doctor referred Clara and her mother for family therapy. Clara was asked what she would like from her mother. She replied, 'Mummy, I want you to stop the rain coming through the roof and into my bedroom, it makes me too sad and scared.' There was no actual leak; Clara's statement was simply a metaphor to say that her very self (the image of the house) was not insulated well enough to protect her from the 'rain' of tears of her mother's grief. When Clara's mother started going to a bereavement counsellor, Clara stopped being agitated and her schoolwork improved dramatically.

Wickes, a Jungian analyst, explains that 'the child's unconscious may be infected by the fears which the mother refuses to recognise as her own' (1988a, p64). In other words, if a parent has a worry, the child will often pick it up and develop a debilitating neurotic symptom around it or even dream about it in order to try to resolve it. This means that children can have the dreams that their parents need to have! When the parent or parents resolve their fears or worries, the child can move on in his own development. Jung, the famous psychoanalyst, made the following statement about this 'participation mystique':

> The 'participation mystique', that is, the primitive unconscious identity of the child with its parents, causes the child to feel the conflicts of the parents, and to suffer from them as if they were its own troubles. It is the things vaguely felt by the child, the oppressive atmosphere of apprehension and self-consciousness, that slowly pervade the child's mind like a poisonous vapour and destroy the security. (Jung, personal communication with Frances Wickes, cited in Wickes, 1988, p57)

Many parents who are unaware of the power of 'participation mystique' will say, 'I won't tell little Johnny that, it will only worry him'. But they do not know that, on some level, little Johnny *already knows*. As Armstrong Perlman (1998, personal communication) says, 'They cannot keep their child from the truth, only the verbalisation of that truth.'

The following examples demonstrate this:

Susan, a young mother was denying to herself the full extent of her grief at a late miscarriage. She tried to 'put it behind her', and to be 'jolly' in front of her five-year old son, Billy. She told Billy that the baby was fine because God was holding him now. The little boy, who until the miscarriage had been perfectly happy, started bed-wetting and repeatedly played hospitals where everyone died. He also had nightmares of overflowing toilets full of poo and tears. When the mother went into therapy and expressed her grief, Billy was fine again and all his symptoms disappeared.

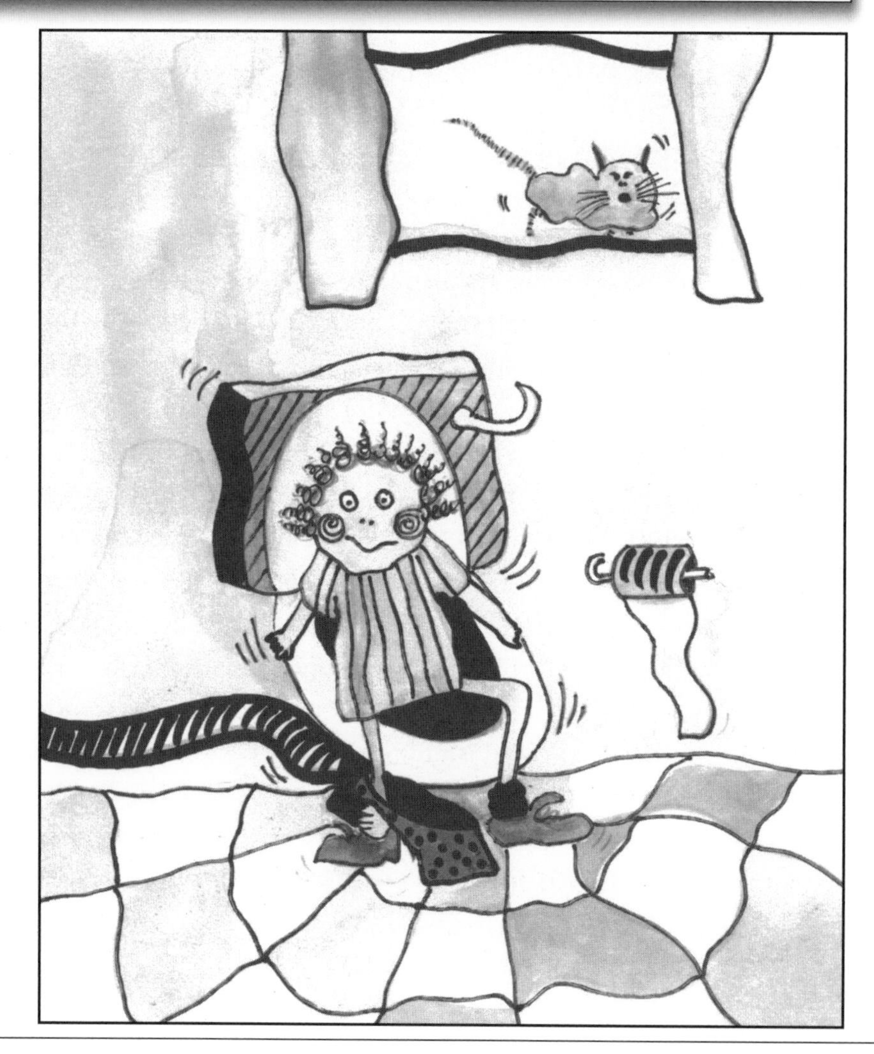

Figure 5
'… and because the toilet wobbled you had to be very careful and hold on tight so you didn't fall in.'

Tessa's mother was trying to keep from her little girl the fact that she had a serious heart complaint and might die. But Tessa said to her teacher, 'Look, I've drawn black holes again for the little girl to fall into.' When the teacher asked why she had fallen in, Tessa said, 'Because she has lost her Mummy. Lost forever, not just for a minute.' Of course, it is totally understandable that a mother would try and protect her child from this horrendous truth, and yet on another level she could not protect her. Tessa's mother couldn't keep her from the truth, only from the verbally expressed truth. Both Tessa and her mother needed professional help, to enable them to talk through and feel their feelings with each other. Without this, Tessa is left holding all her fear and sadness all on her own.

Some anxious children develop obsessive-compulsive rituals, because they are sensing some of their parents' raw, undigested, unprocessed feelings. In developing ordering or checking rituals, they are trying to 'tidy up' mother's too messy feelings. In such cases, the mother really needs to find counselling or psychotherapy for herself. Saying to herself, 'Little Johnny won't pick it up' is simply denial, or grossly inaccurate wishful thinking.

The importance of distinguishing natural, imaginary childhood fears from neurotic ones

This guidebook would not be complete without mentioning the fact that, around the age of four to five, a child's imagination is particularly vivid and strong. For some children, this developmental stage can bring with it waves of fear. For example, when a child is four, the big black wardrobe may indeed appear to be moving towards him in the night, or the face in the curtains be seen as staring cruelly just at him. And when he has a nasty encounter with a table-leg, fridge door, toilet seat or wasp, he can easily feel that it is 'out to get him'. Furthermore, compulsive rituals are common ways through which three-to-five-year-olds manage their anxieties that are strengthened by their often too vivid imaginings. (Think of children who do not dare to step on the pavement cracks, or who check for monsters under the bed each night; or who deal with frightening situations or people by hiding, avoiding, running away or pretending to be ill.)

But if, at this vivid imagination stage, the child also has a very anxious parent, that parent may fail to help the child to transform his sometimes frightening world back into a benign, safe place. Rather, the child may be left with his impressions of the world as menacing or attacking. In contrast, if a child is given consistently a response of empathy and calmness in the face of such paranoid fears, it is far more difficult to keep up a perception of the world as frightening, however vivid his imagination!

> Mother is a real magician, able to [change] the malevolent beings and their little victim. The fire no longer is bad, and the table no longer can hurt. Mother has 'arranged everything'. (Odier, 1956, p90)

Yet, without a soothing mother at this age, a child's ways of coping with anxiety can get stuck, developmentally speaking, at about the age of four; he can sustain all the irrational 'magical thinking' associated with this age-group. For some children, this can endure right into their adulthood, developing into a full-blown neurosis of phobias, obsessions or paranoia.

Children who are wobbly because they have lived in an upside-down world, at home or at school

> Alice thought she had never seen such a curious croquet-ground in her life; it was all ridges and furrows; the balls were live hedgehogs, the mallets live flamingos, and the soldiers had to double themselves up and to stand on their hands and feet, to make the arches. (Lewis Carroll, *Alice in Wonderland*, 1994, p87)

Some homes are 'nonsense' because there are all sorts of negative, highly charged feelings in the air, whereas only 'nice' feelings are being overtly expressed. Others are nonsense homes because a parent is kind and warm one minute, and then cruel and hostile the next. Some homes are nonsense because the child has had to navigate his parents' unpredictable behaviour, to navigate with minimum 'storm damage' their outbreaks of temper, madness, criticism, hostility, depressed moods and so on. Some parents' 'nonsense' comes out in giving the child contradictory messages of 'Come here, I love you' and, the next minute, 'I wish you'd never been born'. Or a child is laughed at and encouraged for his behaviour one day, then punished for doing exactly the same thing the next day. Some children are brought up on an endless diet of chaotic family dramas. Although this can be highly stimulating and very exciting, there is often a lack of anyone with a calm, soothing, still energy in such families. The children therefore have trouble ever feeling calm and still in themselves.

Some 'nonsense homes' are so crazy-making that the child decides he prefers the oasis of his own company. Being with other people is too closely associated with feeling wobbly or agitated inside.

Angela, aged fifteen

We always had to be very quiet when my father was around at home, because of his terrible temper. But sometimes he'd come out of his study and have a really rough-and-tumble game with us all, with lots of shouting (he'd be the loudest), but then all of a sudden, for no apparent reason, he'd switch into being cross and say we were being inconsiderate, and we'd be back to the tiptoeing and Mum going 'Ssshh!' It was so confusing.

One woman remembered being told by her mother as a little girl that she must stop jumping around as she would disturb the people who lived below. They lived in a first-floor apartment above an empty shop. The little girl tried to figure out how she could disturb people *who weren't there*. She was not old enough to place the irrationality firmly at her mother's door. Such homes can closely resemble the sort of places in Lewis Carroll's *Alice in Wonderland*, Edward Lear's nonsense poems or Kafka's persecutory worlds.

Some schools are 'nonsense', upside-down places too, because they attack the expression of tender emotion as weak rather than brave; because bullying is punished in children, but allowed in teachers; because there are rules about keeping off the grass or wearing the right socks but no rules about being unkind to other children. Some teachers choose a job that is all to do with children when they do not like children.

Children from 'nonsense homes' or 'nonsense schools' often try to make sense of the nonsense – to find the logic in it where there is none, and to see as normal what is completely bizarre or abnormal. Trying to make sense out of nonsense can be very taxing and isolating. Alice, for example, in her Wonderland, keeps trying to make sense out of nonsense, and is very lonely because she is trying to do this all on her own.

All nonsense questions are unanswerable. How many hours are there in a mile? Is yellow square or round? (Carroll, 1994, pp58–59)

The jury eagerly wrote down all three dates on their slates, and then added them up, and reduced the answer to shillings and pence. (Carroll, 1994, p120)

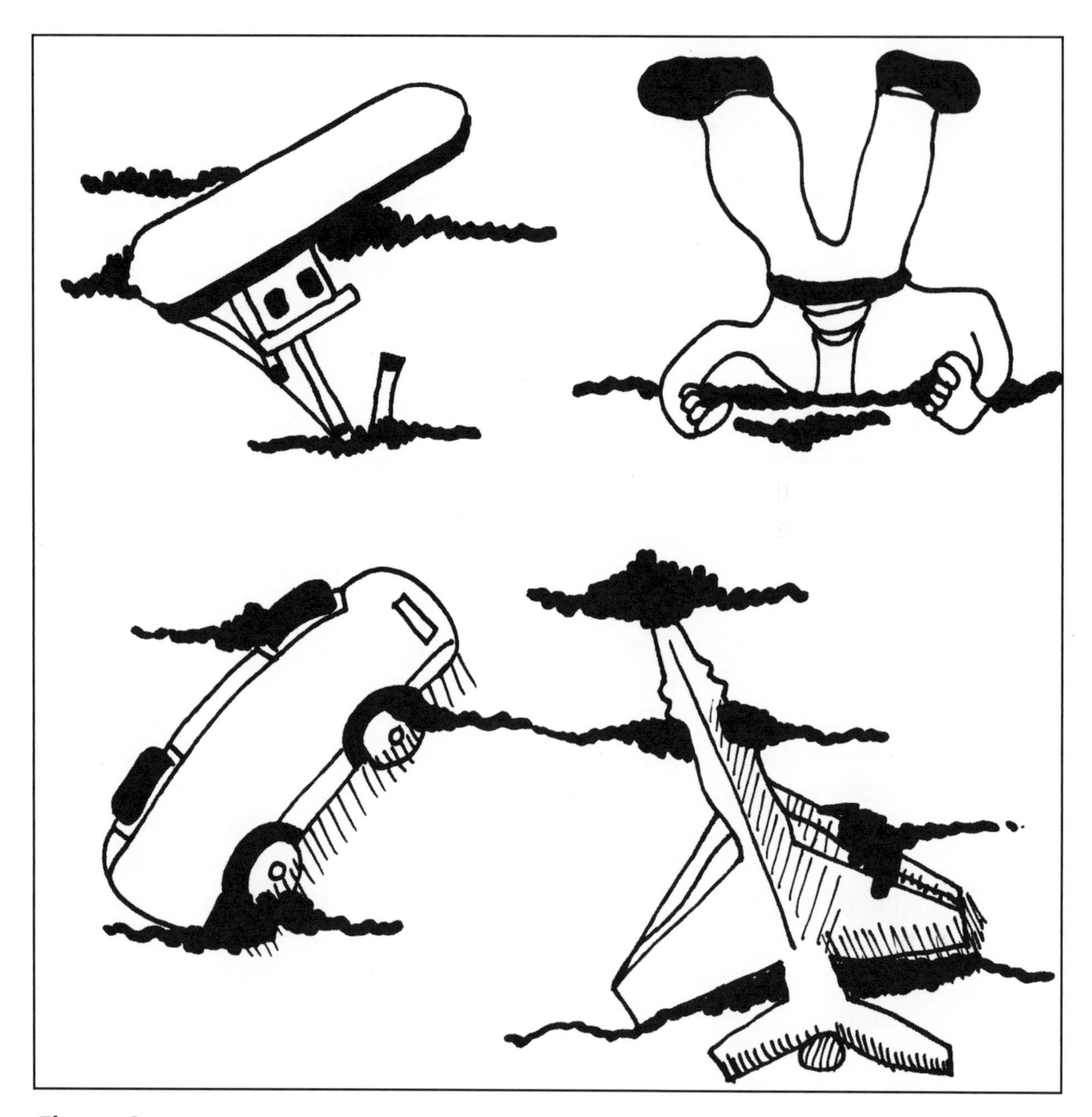

Figure 6
A drawing of a sandplay story about an upside-down world

Not only does the world not seem to make sense to the child, but, worse, he can feel that he does not make sense to himself. Thinking ever harder, 'If I can just think about this some more, I will understand it', he can blame his own lack of comprehension skills and come to believe that it is he who is mad.

The following are stories told by children who are trying to work through their feelings of living in an upside-down, wobbly world:

Mattie, aged nine

Mattie's mother is alcoholic, and is given to sudden explosions. In counselling, Mattie said, 'I'm not scared of anything.' Two minutes later she said, 'I'm scared of everything.' Mattie wrote the following story: 'Sometimes, if you walk across the grass, the grass giant will make the earth scream so loudly that it will pierce your eardrums. But sometimes, if you walk across the grass, there is no grass giant and it's fine. But this means that you can never know anything for sure.'

Billy, aged six

Billy's mother has a drug problem. Billy's siblings are glue-sniffers and go on the streets to steal. Billy's father keeps leaving and coming back. Billy is on the Child Protection Register for Neglect. Billy wrote the following story: 'There are octopuses coming in the house, dustbins are flying through the windows and knocking everything over. A baby is hiding in the wardrobe. It is crying. Someone rings the police for help. But the police fall into the pond and are drowned on the way there. The next day the lollipop lady falls asleep on the job, so the children get run over.'

In other stories of his, little cars regularly fell off the toy garage and people regularly fell out of the doll's house windows. Billy found it terribly difficult and anxiety provoking to move from the classroom to the therapy room, or from the therapy room to the classroom. It was as if he was frightened of falling off the edge of both of them.

David, aged seven

David's mother had died when he was very small. His father then had a string of girlfriends. He would often get engaged and then break it off at the last moment, or break it off after a year of marriage.

In his stories, David had endless couples sitting on benches in a 'Playmobil™' park: 'Dad and me', 'Dad with my real Mum who is dead', 'Dad with a Mum who hasn't arrived yet', 'Dad with a new girlfriend', 'Dad with the girlfriend he's just ditched.'

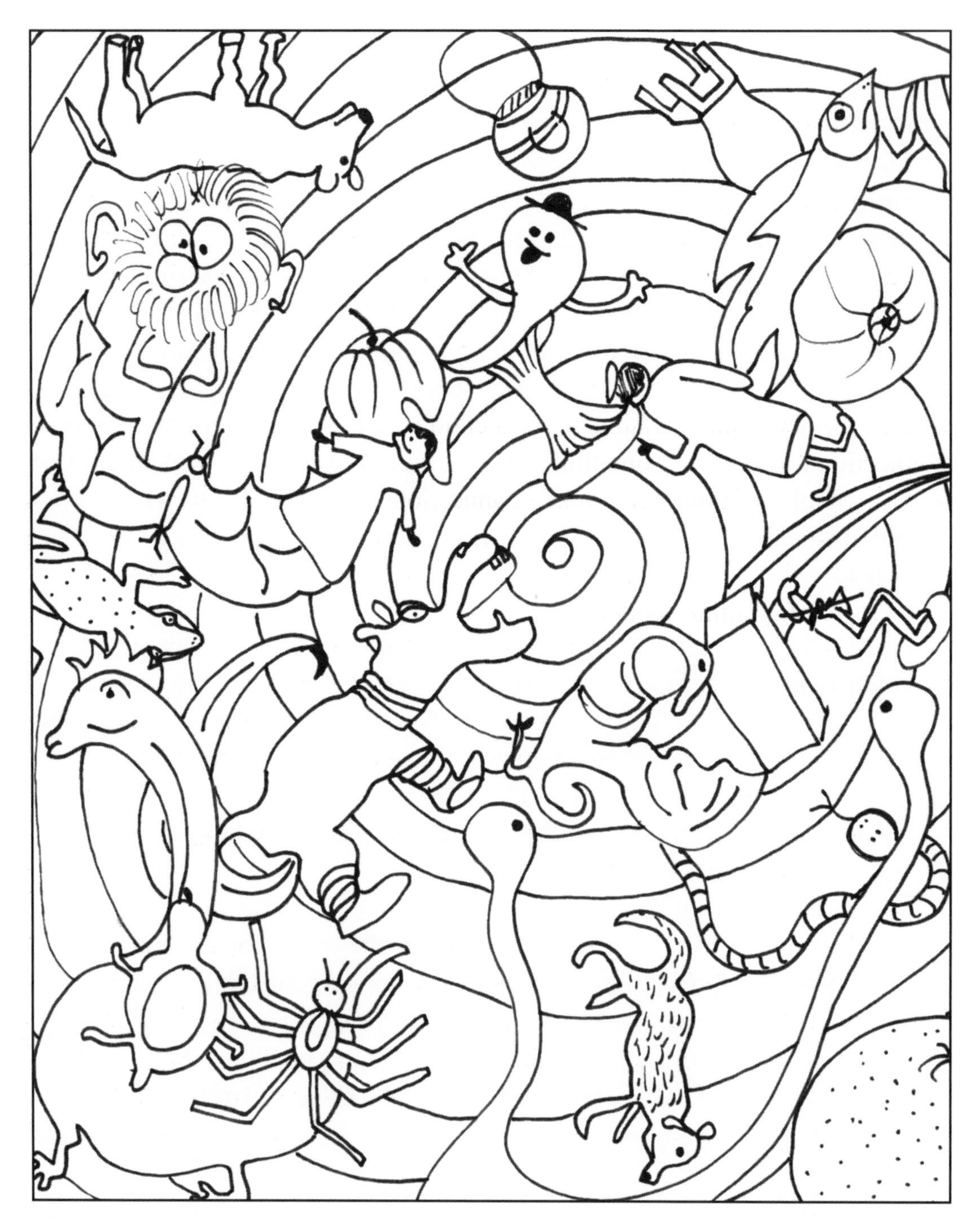

Figure 7 A picture of a story told by a boy about a mass of 'muddly chaos feelings' inside him. He came from a nonsense home.

Children who are wobbly because they have suffered a major trauma that has never been worked through

If a child has suffered a major trauma in his life, and never been helped to fully work through his feelings about it, this can leave a residue of deep anxiety. It is as if the trauma has turned everything upside down for him. So now he is living as if on very shaky ground, waiting for the next volcano, crash, earthquake or meteor, metaphorically speaking.

This occurs not only on a psychological level, but on a biochemical level. For many children suffering from post-traumatic stress, the body-mind keeps pumping out too much stress hormone (cortisol). The effect of this hormone is to tell the brain that there is an emergency, a threat, when there is not. It is like living in a state of hyper-alertness. It robs the child of any possibility of inner peace. The child suffering from post-traumatic stress is usually very wobbly inside, even if he is doing well at covering it up on the outside.

Things are particularly traumatic for a child when a very important emotional connection to someone, something or some part of his life gets broken in some way. Examples of traumatic broken connections are given below, which if not worked through can lead the child to suffer from major anxieties:

Death of a family member.

A parent leaving.

Parents divorcing.

Parents regularly arguing, in frightening or anxiety-making ways.

Witnessing parental violence.

A bankruptcy, or other incident that shook the whole family.

A parent getting 'broken' in some way, as with mental breakdown, depression or serious illness.

Being physically or sexually abused. (If someone who is supposed to be protecting you then abuses you, there is automatically a broken emotional connection.)

A very important relationship that was 'broken' in some way and was never repaired or re-established.

The following are some of the most common symptoms when a child is suffering from post-traumatic stress (adapted from the *Diagnostic and Statistical Manual of Mental Disorders*, 4th edn, 1994, American Psychiatric Association, p428):

Agitated behaviour.

Recurrent recollections of the traumatic event (in young children, repetitive play in which themes or aspects of the trauma are expressed).

Recurrent distressing dreams of the event.

Acting or feeling as if the traumatic event were recurring.

Distress at events that symbolise or resemble an aspect of the traumatic event.

Efforts to avoid thoughts, feelings, activities and situations associated with the trauma.

In young children loss of recently acquired developmental skills, such as toilet training or language skills.

Restricted range of feeling (for example, unable to have loving feelings).

Sleeping problems.

Feeling detached from people.

Concentration problems, loss of interest in things previously found interesting.

Being tense and on guard.

Angry outbursts or irritability.

Whether or not traumatic events leave the child with a legacy of too difficult levels of stress and anxiety like this will depend principally on two things. First, was someone emotionally 'there' for the child after the event, someone who was emotionally available enough to help the child to express and deal with his feelings about what happened? This is not a question of a 'one-off' experience of listening, but of someone being there, over time, while the child works through his roller-coaster of different feelings about the event, one by one, as they surface. It needs to be someone who is not frightened by the emotional intensity of fully expressed, fully felt emotional pain, shock, fear and loss. Otherwise, they are likely to block the child's emotional processing and his coming to terms with the event.

Second, did someone explain to the child what happened, or did they keep the child in the dark, in a state of confusion, fear and ignorance? Parents who believe 'Best not to tell him about what happened', or 'Best not to let him say good-bye to his father who has just died, he's too young', or 'Best put it behind us now, for his sake', are actually 'stacking the dice' for that child to lead a life of feeling too anxious. It is often because parents are unable to handle their own feelings that they assume that the child is unable to handle his. But they often do not give him a chance. For example, Daddy walks out one day and never comes back. If the child does not have someone emotionally available and receptive enough for him to deal with his feelings of anger, grief, betrayal, rejection, worthlessness, guilt and so on, and if he is kept in the dark, this child is heading for a great deal of neurotic suffering in later life. If he cannot voice his feelings to someone who can really listen, he is left holding them all by himself.

Bowlby, a leading psychoanalyst in the field of childhood trauma, found in his research (1978) that those people still suffering in adulthood from the effects of a trauma in childhood, were those who had not had the benefit of the principal requirements identified above.

Child counselling or therapy can stop the painful effects of post-traumatic stress or unprocessed trauma. With counselling or therapy, the 'emotional circuitry [in the brain] can be re-educated' (Goleman, 1996, p208).

UNDERSTANDING WHAT LIFE IS LIKE FOR CHILDREN LIKE JOE

Why some children like Joe long for wobbles, muddles or messes

> *Fox:* Do you enjoy all this flummery, Mr Pitt?
> *Pitt:* No, Mr Fox.
> *Fox:* Do you enjoy anything, Mr Pitt?
> *Pitt:* A balance sheet, Mr Fox. I enjoy a good balance sheet.
> (Bennett, *The Madness of King George,* 1995, p8)

For a child like Joe, life can seem just too rigid, tidy and predictable. He can long to break out and let go. He can long for some chaos, some disorder, as if thereby to re-establish a balance inside himself. The order in his life can seem to strangle everything spontaneous and free in him. It can bring its own boredom too, stripping major experiences of their intensity and excitement. And yet, try as he might, Joe cannot seem to loosen up. He cannot give up his need to feel in control, despite its stranglehold of anti-life and anti-fun.

Children like Joe do not jump up or down with joy; do not roll down grassy banks, do not use exuberant words like 'Yippee!'; or say 'Hey, let's do X or Y!!'. They do not feel wildly passionate about someone or something. By and large, children like Joe have only well controlled feelings.

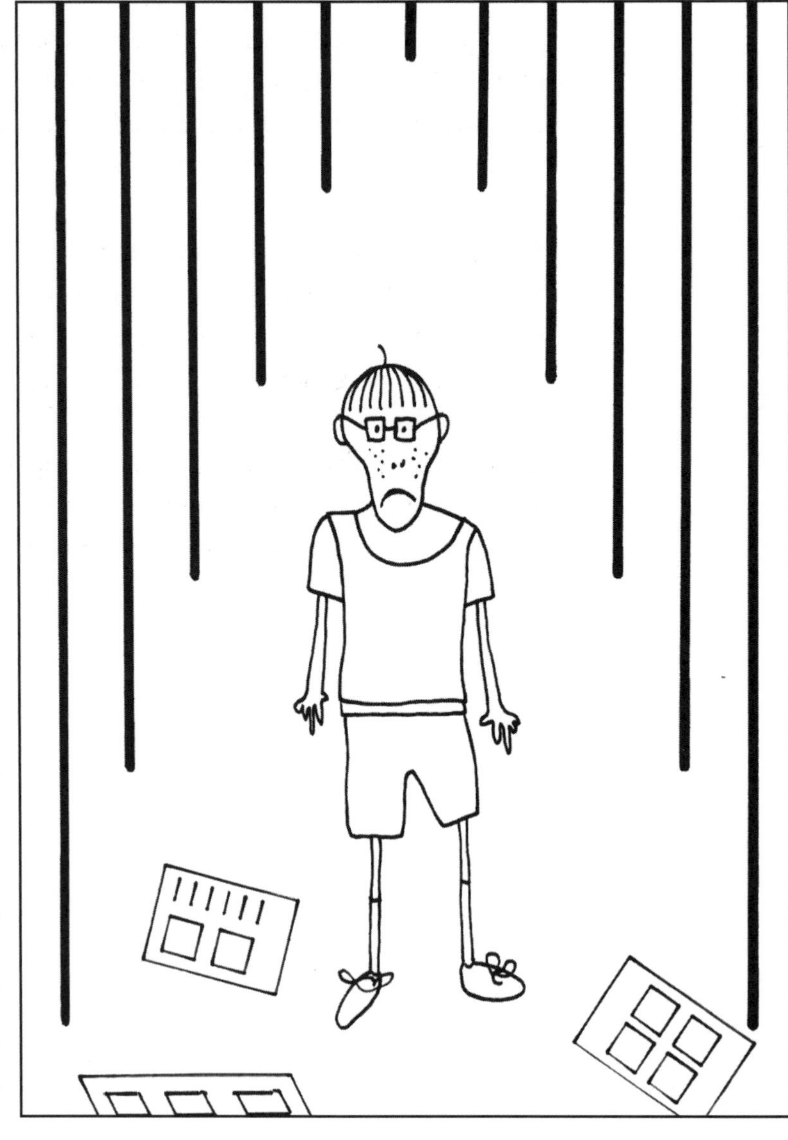

Figure 8 All about Joe

Some children like Joe find it difficult to play make-believe, or to join in rough-and-tumble play. Rather, they tend to play nicely with board games, puzzles or computers. Sometimes children like Joe can be so tightly held-in that they can make people in their company lose their spontaneity and creativity too. In fact, the sad thing is that people often find children like Joe just too dull. He himself may also believe this is all he is.

He may watch other children playing and wish dearly to be like them, as if maybe some of their spontaneity and unselfconscious happiness might 'rub off' on to him. A child like Joe often knows on some level that he is missing out on far too much. He is indeed missing out on too many of life's riches: the life of the body, of the imagination, of carefree play, of passionate engagement, of the sensual, of letting go into intense states of anxiety-free pleasure. He is missing out on all the amazing things that can happen from going with the unpredictable, the spontaneous, the moment of inspiration and creative risk. Of course, creativity is born of chaos, and not order. 'The tragedy of life is not so much what men suffer, but rather what they miss' (Carlyle, cited in Auden & Kronenberger, 1964, p18).

How some children like Joe live in their head instead of their heart or their body

Many children like Joe have found a way to cut themselves off from much of their feeling life and the life of their body, as (on a conscious or unconscious level) they find strong feelings far too dangerous. So they choose to live in their heads. Living in their heads gives such children an illusion of control. They can try to reason everything out. They can try to think themselves out of their troublesome feelings.

Many children like Joe do not enjoy their body because, rather than it being a source of pleasure, it is a source of anxiety. It is as if the body is somehow a separate and slightly maverick entity with a will of its own. It might do something embarrassing, or lose control in some shameful way. It is in this vein that Milner, a psychotherapist, describes a patient who was 'deeply musical but can hardly listen to concerts for fear that she will scream or perhaps wet herself' (1987, p124).

How some children like Joe fear the threat of too much life

> We can only recognise that [life force] is absent and that anxiety is observed in its place. (Freud, 1917)

Children like Joe often have a belief (usually out of their conscious awareness) that, if they were to let themselves really feel what they feel, the whole thing could get terrifyingly out-of-control. Passionate engagement in life feels like such an out-of-control affair. 'What if you start crying and you cannot stop? What if you get angry and became a volcano?' There is often an underlying fear of becoming overwhelmed in some way: consumed by feeling, flooded by it. So children like Joe tend to guard against intense emotional states such as anger, excitement, love or intense states of need or desire. Order in some form or another is used to fend off the threat of any such intensity. Moreover, selectivity in terms of choosing which emotions to feel, and which to try not to feel, simply does not work. If you cut yourself off from intense feelings such as anger, fear or grief, it usually means you have difficulty feeling intense positive arousal states as well, such as delight, exhilaration, excitement or love.

When a child like Joe feels threatened by too-strong feelings, he will try to use order, thinking or reason so that he can have 'little' feelings – manageable ones, rather than big ones. But, as Blume says, 'What passes for order is really frozen chaos' (1990, p34). With these children, it is the frozen chaos of too many held-in feelings.

But it is a tragic thing to be frightened of strong feelings like this, because strong feelings are about life-force; about feeling truly and intensely alive; about the capacity for powerful, profound or intensely nourishing connection to someone. Moreover, passionate feelings are essential for making dreams come true. So the price of trying not to feel too much life is often far too high. Commonly, it is a price of dullness and blandness for too much of the time. It means life can lose too much of its meaning. Moreover, the child can present as dull or boring, sometimes robotic: 'I may only have a little life, but at least I am in control of it' (an adolescent, self-confessed computer addict).

How some children like Joe use order or obsessive-compulsive behaviour to try to ward off their too strong feelings

> Dear me. Most interesting. Evidently you're quite one of us. Not so far gone as me, of course. Otherwise you wouldn't dare relax for one moment. With me, if once the hair weren't accurately combed, the shoes properly laced, every object exactly placed, the same bus caught every morning, *The Times* always carried under the left arm, the entire structure would collapse. (White, 1979, p316)

Children like Joe often do things like touching all the railings on the way home, washing their hands a lot, counting things, avoiding things, checking things, repeating things. Obsessive behaviour is one way in which both adults and children try to stop themselves having the feelings they are having: compulsive rituals, such as checking something when you have already checked it several times, washing your hands again and again, refusing to ever walk on a crack in the pavement.

Compulsive rituals give the child some sense that he is warding off an awful danger, but this is called 'magical thinking', as he is fending off a threat he perceives in his outer world, when in fact the real danger lies in his inner world, in the form of his own intense emotional arousal. Consider the following example:

Philip, aged ten

Philip had a compulsion to lock doors. He could not sleep at night until he had checked at least six times that the front door was locked. When he stopped 'locking out of himself' all his grief about his mother's death, and then cried and cried, he no longer had this compulsion with doors.

As Rycroft says, 'Feelings come to be regarded as intruders which disturb the orderliness of the world of which the obsessional has made himself master' (1988, p77). So compulsive rituals can make children like Joe feel in control, when underneath they usually feel anything but 'in control'. Rituals mean that at least you are doing something to feel in control when you or your world feels so threateningly out of control.

Nasrudin was throwing handfuls of crumbs around his house.
'What are you doing?' someone asked him.
'Keeping the tigers away.'
'But there are no tigers in these parts.'
'That's right. Effective, isn't it?' (Shah, 1966, p20)

For a child battling with feelings of intense anxiety, the ritual can make him feel 'gathered in'. The ritual can bind the anxiety. It is a last-ditch attempt to try to make the world feel safe. But the child's obsessive behaviour may drive the people in his life to distraction. Relatives or teachers often do not see the fear behind the desperate need for order and control. They often feel only the frustration with the time wasting: 'Sorry, but we can't leave yet. Adam [aged eight] needs to touch all the windows before he goes out.'

How some children like Joe are worryingly good

Some children like Joe look too tidy, speak too tidily, go about their business with the utmost correctness. They may generally behave like 'little adults'. Some children like Joe are just far too good. Unfortunately, they are often mistaken for being 'contented', or well adjusted and well behaved. The truth is that often they are cut off from too much of their life-force.

Some 'too good' children are trying so hard to be perfect that they can hardly breathe for fear of making a mistake. They give mistakes 'disaster' status. They have linked mistakes with failure, humiliation, shame or the withdrawal of love or approval. Some 'too good' children cannot stop studying and let themselves go into pleasure because they believe that they are loved for what they achieve or do in life more than for who they are. Playing, messing about, just being or daring to be naughty may, in their minds, threaten this love.

Understanding why children like Joe cannot let go

Some childhood homes are too concerned with tidiness and straight lines, and not enough with play, fun and sensual pleasure.

I'd had a spotlessly sanitised childhood, with a change of Aertex support systems every other day . . . I had been a wanted, planned for, waited for, only child, a fully rounded 'gooseberry' to a devoted couple. In those days I'd had plans as well. One of these plans was to extend this safe sanitised childhood indefinitely. (Cook, 1991, p28)

Some children like Joe come from a home environment that is too tidy, too clean and too regulated with too high standards. An adult from a childhood background like this said, 'When I was a child my mother was far more passionate about tidying than she was about me.' Some childhood homes like this are full of unquestioned, formal rituals and spoken or unspoken house rules about 'the proper way to do things' or 'the things that just aren't done'. The child may have been brought up with very tight codes of behaviour, and very rigid thinking about what is right and wrong. This tends to stifle impulses to play, laugh and generally have fun.

> These adults are essentially too adult and their often very effective parenting causes their child to follow too quickly and too completely in their footsteps. That which is childlike, animal-like, passionate, sensual, or self-indulgent is kept under tight control. These forces are harnessed, and the child is taught that this is the way to be. (Johnson, 1994, p275)

Such families can be described by a line from the film, *If Walls Could Talk*: 'Could you throw away your morals just for one minute and help me?' In families like this, you can often find 'excited heads' with too little life of the body – that is, very minimal affectionate touch or physical expression of love. After babyhood, the child may have been sensually deprived, meaning too few cuddles, too few experiences of the pleasure of skin on skin, skin in water, on sand, in sun. In short, children like Joe do not live in a sensual world.

Tony, aged nine

Tony was a very uptight little boy who preferred to read books than to go out at playtime with other children. Teachers were worried about him, as he seemed to live totally in his head. On holiday, on the beach Tony's father felt too uncomfortable taking off his shirt, or his shoes and socks. He found it very difficult to touch Tony. In fact, he felt no real desire to do so. No one had ever really cuddled Tony, picked him up and carried him around. There was no enjoyment of skin on skin in his house.

So children like Joe who come from such backgrounds have often had too few significant adults in their life to teach them about letting go, fun, pleasure and how to play. If an adult can play well; if he or she can easily enjoy imaginative, fun or sensual play, this is a sign of emotional health. Maslow, a psychotherapist, dedicated much of his life to the study of happy, fulfilled, emotionally healthy people. These are some of his conclusions:

> The most mature people are the ones that can have the most fun. These people can regress at will, can become childish and play with children and be close to them . . . It is becoming more and more apparent that what we call a normal adult adjustment involves turning one's back on what would threaten us. And what does threaten us is softness, fantasy, emotion, 'childishness'. (Maslow, 1971, pp82–3; 89)

In short, if a child has parents who cannot play, be spontaneous or physically affectionate, that child may never really have a childhood in any real sense of the word.

How children can get to be like Joe if their teachers or parents could not cope with anything less than total compliance

> And before you let the sun in, mind it wipes its shoes. (Dylan Thomas, 1995, p338)

Some 'far too good' children, or children who cannot let go, have been trained out of their stronger, freer feelings, leaving them feeling deadened in their inner world – and maybe not knowing why. The problem is that life and passion can be locked away so deeply inside that it can be very difficult to find them again. In fact, many such children forget they ever had intense feelings (particularly if these feelings were repressed in babyhood). They think that the nice, compliant self that they present to the world is who they really are, is all there is. As a little girl aged eight said, 'All I feel is dull, I know it's because I'm dull. It's just how I am.'

Some children kill off much of their passion and life-force, in order to keep their parents' love and approval for them alive. Hence the tragic paradox for so many children that, to feel loved, they must only live a partial version of themselves. Where there is a strong attachment between parent and child, it is unbearable for a child to think of losing that parent's love. This love is his air, his oxygen, his raison d'être, the very basis of his self-esteem.

Some parents or teachers simply cannot cope with a child as a fully alive child, a child with a wide range of emotions, a child who wants to express these emotions spontaneously and passionately (which can mean loudly). Such parents or teachers often cannot cope, because their child's exuberance is too much of a contrast to how deadened *they* feel. In their own childhood, it may have been that states of high emotion such as excitement, anger or protest were unacceptable, unresponded to, or responded to in a shaming or frightening way.

One father realised in therapy that his own mother had squeezed the life out of him, because she was so strict; so now, unaware, he was doing this to his own children. Anything remotely resembling life (such as excitement, noise, mess, or glee) in his children he criticised heavily. He could not bear to see in them the life he had killed off in himself. It can indeed be very painful for such adults to see children living to the full, and expressing the feelings which they have stifled in themselves. So sometimes a fully expressive child can provoke envy (usually unconscious or denied) in their parents or teachers. As a result, some parents or teachers start finding 'reasons' to justify why natural, passionately expressed feelings in the child are not OK. So squeals of delight, jumping up and down with joy, very loud crying or raging are viewed as 'bad', 'naughty', a 'threat to their discipline', 'inconsiderate to the neighbours', 'getting over-excited', with the conclusion that 'I'm a weak parent or teacher if I don't squash this right now.' For some adults, it would be too awful to acknowledge the full extent of their own, unlived passion. It can be far simpler to justify the view that it is 'in the child's best interests' to be criticised, scorned or shamed into feeling he is being too noisy, hyperactive or out of control.

Children who are with adults such as these can easily feel shamed. This usually means the child will rein in his expressiveness and his expansiveness. He may retreat to the safety of a world of 'thinking' that *is* acceptable to the adults in his life, and then the slow fading of the full richness of his character.

Lizzie, aged ten

Before Lizzie went into counselling, she was a lifeless kind of child. She just got on with her school work, but never got excited about anything. Lizzie can remember how, at four years old, she had pretended to be a champion rower in a boat (the bath). She said to her mother, 'Look at me! See, I'm a champion rower!' She recalls how her mother had punished her for 'showing-off', and 'being noisy and inconsiderate'. Lizzie remembers regular, similar scolding for laughing; for being loudly delighted; for jumping up and down with joy. She also remembers making mudpies as a love gift for her mother. Her mother told her to take them back to the garden at once, because of the dirt and mess in her kitchen. When Lizzie cried, her father called her a wimp and said, 'Where's my big strong girl gone?' Lizzie had learnt to adjust to the narrow range of feeling states that were acceptable to her mother and father. The price she paid for her parents' approval was to stifle far too much in herself.

How different it might have been, had Lizzie's mother shared her *joie de vivre* and received her daughter's love graciously. How different, if her father could have stayed with Lizzie's hurt and sadness, listened and comforted her *through* it, not *out of* it.

In counselling, Lizzie's fully expressive self started to emerge after she realised that her counsellor was not going to respond like her parents. Her passion came out in her dreams and her art, through images of floods and earthquakes and radiant colour. As her counsellor encouraged her life, rather than suffocated it, she began to be able to live it. But Lizzie was smart. At home she put away her 'life', and just brought it out at school and with her friends. Home reported 'no change'. School reported 'amazing change'. 'It's as if she's been unlocked,' her teachers said.

> The more one-sided a society's observance of strict moral principles such as orderliness, cleanliness . . . and the more deep-seated its fear of the other side of human nature – vitality, spontaneity, sensuality, critical judgement and inner independence – the more strenuous will be its efforts to isolate this hidden territory, to surround it with silence or institutionalise it. Prostitution, the pornography trade, and almost obligatory obscenity typical of traditionally all-male groups such as the military are part of the legalised, even requisite, reverse side of this cleanliness and order. (Miller, 1990, p192)

How children can present as dull or deadened because they have simply not met enough life

> In the afternoons my mother and father both retired to sleep. That is, they retired to death. They really died for the afternoons. (Alvarez, 1971, p148)

When children repeatedly complain of boredom at home or at school, some are communicating about something too dead in the atmosphere, or too deadened in their teachers or parents. Some children who present as dull have had too many sterile, formal or over serious interactions with the adults in their lives. Some school or home atmospheres can be sensed as soon as you walk into them. The air feels joyless and heavy, with no sense of play: sometimes like a courtroom; sometimes like a morgue; sometimes like a strict convent, sometimes with all the sterility of a scrubbed-clean hospital –

sensually dead. Some atmospheres are heavily laden with guilt and shame. In other cases the air is stale from too many cold silences. Some are thick with a bleakness from there having been all too few warm and tender exchanges in a long time. Sometimes there is something too dead in the parents' relationship. Sometimes depression hangs in the atmosphere.

Young children, still in the process of forming a self, are unfortunately too open to such atmospheres: so much so that they can become a dead weight inside them, get in their blood so to speak, become a part of their way of being in the world. Often the more the parents are denying their own feelings, the heavier the weight for their child.

Max (adolescent) who says he feels trapped inside himself

I wish as a child I could have said to my mother, 'Mummy, your depression was not a little thing. Not only did it leak right through the house, it became my deadness'.

Sally (adolescent)

Sally had been a very serious, far too good little girl. When she was 16, she went into therapy for major depression. Sally's father always presented as 'I'm just fine', but underneath he was living with too much defeat from his own childhood. He had killed off much of his passion to survive his own frightening father. Sally sensed it. In therapy, Sally said, 'It's the death trapped inside me that is so frightening, not the life.'

However, it is important to say, that some children are saved from imbibing the deadness of others by finding someone in their life who, consistently and repeatedly over time, offers them warm, expansive and very alive contact. Sometimes this is an aunt, or a friendly neighbour, or a good nanny or teacher. But this must be someone with whom the child has regular contact. Fleeting or occasional enlivened interactions with such people are not enough to transport or inspire children like Joe into another way of being. The real tragedy is when a child like Joe has no such person in his childhood. As Rowan says, 'We may choose to grow, to stagnate, or to decline, and in a world where there is little encouragement to grow, most of us may not do it very much or at all' (1986, p13).

The powerful, unconscious communication from parent to child about the danger of strong feelings

> Somewhere along the way, I learnt to just have nice little feelings. (Charles, aged 14)

Sometimes there is a powerful, 'underground', unconscious communication from parent to child about the 'dangerous' nature of strong feelings. Some parents who fear the 'threatening mess' of their own intense feelings often move into controlling mode. This includes controlling their children's time, space, beliefs, feelings and wants: 'No, you don't feel this, you feel that', 'No, you want this, not that.' Parents who are defending against their own feelings in this way can find the strongly expressed emotions (such as distress or exuberance) in their babies or children most disturbing, because they are so frightened of their own feelings getting out of control.

The child's alive feelings meet something too threatened in his parent. For this reason, some parents find their child's untidiness just awful, as it triggers a fear of being overwhelmed by mess. But what they are often so threatened by on an unconscious level, is their own internal mess, the mess of too many bottled up, unprocessed, undigested feelings. These are often projected via an absolute over-reaction to and abhorrence of a child's messy bedroom. As one parent said, 'Billy's toys all over the kitchen floor make me want to scream. A single jam stain on the door can send me into rage. It makes my blood boil . . . I know it's not rational, but . . . ' Many such children then, sadly, internalise their parent's obsessive need for tidiness.

Children are very vulnerable to the emotional inhibitions of the adults in their lives, both parents and teachers. So if these adults block their own feelings of anger, excitement or joy, their own capacity to be spontaneous, free or impulsive, sadly these rich colours of humanness may remain unevoked, unborn in the child, either partially or in a major way. It is in this sense that Ann Alvarez (a child psychotherapist) talks of the 'undrawn child' (1992; 1997) as opposed to the 'withdrawn' child.

Many family belief systems with a lot of 'Don't feel', or 'Don't feel that', non-verbal messages are passed down from one generation to another. Family belief systems can, for example, cause one generation of girls after another to cut themselves off from their more masculine qualities in order to accommodate to family norms, which want them to be pretty (that is, decorative), but not powerful. Similarly, boys may be encouraged to kill off their feminine qualities, and then be unable to feel tender, loving feelings.

Obsessive behaviour and over-ordering as a way of trying to live life

With compulsive rituals and overt ordering, the reasoning usually goes something like this: 'If I try to order something in my outer world, I can feel more in control in my inner world.' The irony is that the more you try to establish external order over inner chaos, the more the inner chaos often builds up pressure. The energetic charge from this pressure leaks out in all manner of neurotic symptoms. Hence the vicious cycle for many children like Joe: the more they try to sit on too strong feelings, the more tight, obsessive or 'straight-line' they can feel.

Some children like Joe have had very wobbly babyhoods, which have left them with too much chaos and wobble and a frightening level of anxiety. They did not receive enough soothing and help with their distress during this time. In childhood they may therefore develop obsessive bevahiour as a way of trying to ward off the too dangerous feelings left from their babyhood. Early patterns of 'self-holding', when a baby is far too young to be able to 'think' through his feelings in any way, can often result in ordering rituals in later life.

When a child like Joe has no one to help him with his emotions that feel just too dangerous, obsessive rituals or similar controlling behaviour can feel like the only way of making the world safe. He has lost faith in anybody's ability to make the world safe for him, so must adopt drastic measures to make the world safe for himself. Some checking rituals engaged in by children are a form of clinging to something, trying to make at least part of the environment predictable, dependable. As one adolescent suffering from checking rituals to do with lights being on or off put it, 'It's like I cling to it, the light bulb, the switch. It soothes me.'

When children are frightened to let go, because they are frightened of someone in their lives

Some children are just too frightened to be fully expressive and spontaneous. You have to feel free inside yourself to be able to be that. If you have a domineering or authoritarian parent or teacher of whom you are frightened, if you have been on the receiving end of too many criticisms, commands or actual abuse, life is far too serious an affair for you to feel free, expansive and expressive. One woman remembered in therapy that, as a little child, a relative would always tell her, 'Go and find your cousin and whatever he's doing, tell him to stop it.' It had always been a family joke, but, over the years, the woman remembered seeing that cousin become more and more withdrawn.

There can be no 'blossoming' in a child whose parent or teacher is constantly being critical, condemning or frightening. Although there may be lots of achievements in their outer life, it is difficult for anything to really flourish in terms of the development of personhood. Some children who have had a frightening parent go on to develop obsessive-compulsive behaviour. They develop rituals to fend off some imaginary danger. This is often an unconscious and displaced attempt to try to ward off some too frightening energy in their parent, as if warding off a 'bad spirit' and stopping it from getting inside.

When a child is held in because he has suffered a trauma

If a child has suffered a major shock or trauma, he may feel that life has gone out of control. Trauma can rock a child's very sense of the world as a safe place, rock any sense of his security in being in the world.

One way in which many children cope with this is to try to impose some sense of order on their outer world, when inside everything feels all shaken up, disturbed and topsy-turvy. An expert on incest survivors notes their frequent 'attempts to control things that don't matter, just to control something' (Blume, 1990, pxix). Hence some children develop obsessive-compulsive rituals after a shock or trauma. Such rituals are an attempt to organise and fix external reality when, in their inner world, everything is all over the place, thrown wide open. This is why, for the child, the successful completion of ordering rituals, without being interrupted by someone trying to hurry them on, can feel like a matter of life or death.

But rituals or compulsive ordering behaviour only offer temporary relief. All too often, without professional help, feelings evoked by the trauma will remain unprocessed and, as long as they are not processed, the neurotic symptoms will persist.

What can happen to children like Joe in later life if they do not get help?

Some children like Joe simply fall into a life of unquestioning conformity, in which the tightness of an over-ordered life becomes an enslaving habit. Others, however, at some stage rebel. For them, being overcontrolled in a family where 'messy' feelings are not allowed can feel so stifling and imprisoning, that at some point, it can provoke them into a major reaction against their emotional straitjacket.

Breaking out of an over-ordered childhood can happen in adolescence, with its often explosive breaking away into independence, rebelling against the system, living with fast-changing hormones and physical change, huge mood swings, crushes, first experiences of sex and so on. Sometimes the threat to the too tightly held-in family status quo reaches a head when the adolescent is seen to experiment with sexuality or drugs. It can blast a family apart. Tragically also in some cases, where order has been holding together a too fragile self, this breaking out can also bring about the adolescent's breakdown.

Some children with a tightly held-in self are drawn to chaos in later life as a counter-force, but the problem is that, in the process, some then overdose on chaos and live too dangerously, as if to make up for lost time, over drinking; dangerous driving; dangerous drug taking; sleeping rough and so on. Others may organise their life so that they find their 'chaos needs' met by having complicated extra-marital affairs where lots of people get hurt, or by being chaotic with money or responsibilities.

WHAT YOU CAN DO AFTER YOU HAVE READ WILLY AND THE WOBBLY HOUSE TO THE CHILD

This section offers ideas for things to say and do after the story *Willy and the Wobbly House* has been read to the child. The tasks, games and exercises are specifically designed to help a child to think about, express and further digest his feelings about the story's emotional theme, which mirrors his own feelings.

Children, as we have said, often cannot speak clearly and fully in everyday language about what they are feeling, but they can show or enact, draw or play out their feelings about it. Therefore, many of the points in this section offer support for creative, imaginative and playful ways of expression. To avoid asking the child too many questions (children can soon feel interrogated), some exercises just require a tick in a box, or the choosing of a word or image from a selection. The tasks, games and exercises are also designed to inspire a child to respond further by telling his own stories.

Please note The tasks, games and exercises are not designed to be worked through in chronological order. Also, there are far too many to attempt them all in one go – the child could feel bombarded. Just pick the ones you think would be right for the child you are working with, taking into account their age and how open they are to the subject matter. Instructions to the child are in tinted boxes.

✳ Feeling like Willy, or feeling like Joe

Do you ever feel like Willy?
When?

____

____

Do you ever feel like Joe?
When?

____

____

✳ The place of feeling good

Willy and Joe felt so much better when they found the Puddle World.

- Draw a real or imaginary place you would like to go to, which you think would make you feel happier or better.
- What would the people in that place be like?
- How would they be with you?
- Where would they take you?
- What would they say to you?

✳ A visit to the Puddle World

- If you could go to the Puddle World, would you rather go to 'Still' or to the 'Giggle Pool'?
- Why?
- What would you do there? Draw it or say it.

✻ Your life as a garden

- If your life was a garden, what sort of garden would it be: overgrown, too neat, with lots of weeds, lots of flowers, nothing growing, too high walls that block out the sun?
- Now draw it.
- What would you like to change in your life as a garden?
- What would you like to stay the same in your life as a garden?

✻ You and your wobbly feelings

Have available paints, Play-Doh®, clay and so on, so that children can actually make a big blobby mess on the paper.

- Show a wobbly jelly-feeling mess on the page.
- How do you feel, now you have done it?
- Do you ever feel like this inside?
- If so, is your feeling inside a bigger mess or a smaller mess than the one on the page?

✻ You and your too tidy feelings

- Now make a very neat-and-tidy shape.
- How do you feel, now you have done it?
- Do you ever feel like this inside?
- If so, do you feel more neat and tidy than the shape you have drawn, or less?

✳ The wobble of worry

When you feel too wobbly, or too worried inside, does it remind you of any of these? Tick any that do, then draw them.

Tangled knitting ☐

A wobbly jelly ☐

A big, messy puddle ☐

Everything happening all at once: like telephones ringing, babies crying, cars hooting, people shouting, dogs barking ☐

Like when you drop what you are carrying and it goes all over the place ☐

Lots of bats or moths flying around far too fast and knocking into things ☐

Something like very thin glass, that could break and crack at any minute ☐

A too messy bedroom when you cannot find what you are looking for ☐

A rubbish bin crammed to the brim ☐

Things in too many pieces ☐

An overgrown garden ☐

Lights flashing really fast ☐

Piles of paper slipping off the table ☐

A demolition site ☐

A storm or hurricane ☐

If none of these are right for you, just draw or write your own image for when you feel the 'wobble of worry' inside you.

✳ The adults in your head

Tick which adults you have in your head from the picture. These are people who you think about quite often, even if you do not really want to spend time thinking about some of them. In your head do you have:

1 A shouting one ☐
2 A kind, gentle one ☐
3 One who seems to like other children more than they like you ☐
4 A delicious, warm one who makes you feel very safe about being in the world ☐
5 A frightening one ☐
6 One who is like the Puddle Queen, who makes you feel all calm and good when you are upset ☐

Which of these people in your head make you more wobbly inside, and which make you feel less wobbly inside?

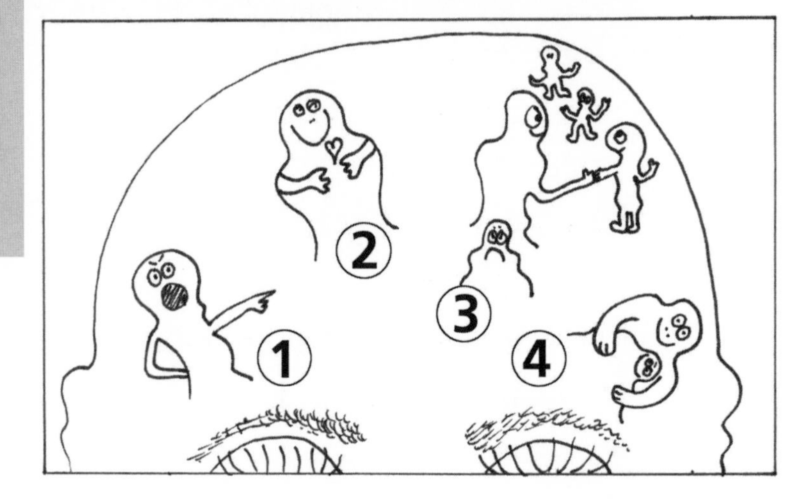

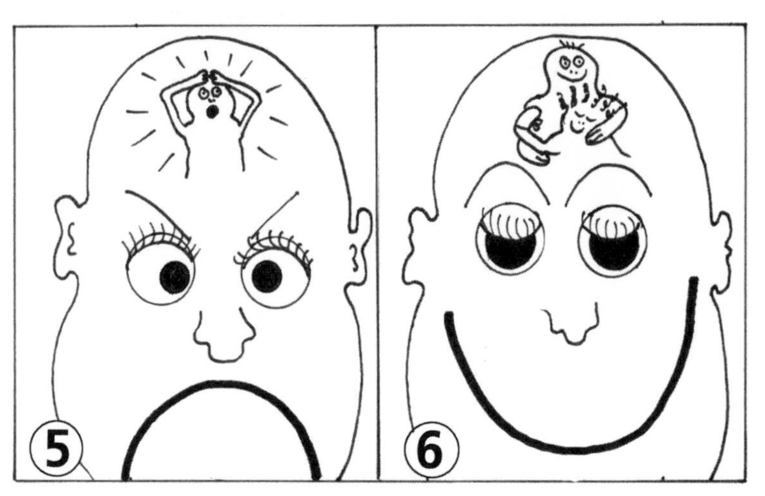

Figure 9
The adults in your head

✻ The wobbly you and the not-wobbly you

- What does it feel like to be you when you are feeling wobbly?
- Make a clay image of it.
- Show the feeling in a movement.
- Play out in music what it feels like.
- Draw a picture of you like this.
- What does it feel like when you are not feeling wobbly inside?
- Make a clay image of it.
- Show the feeling in a movement.
- Play out in music what it feels like.
- Draw a picture of you feeling good inside, not wobbly.

✳ Feelings without names

The following exercise helps children describe their strong, nameless feelings, which can feel far more threatening because they are nameless.

- Do you have some feelings that worry you because you don't know what they are, or because you don't have names for them? If you have some of these nameless feelings, draw what it feels like inside you when you have them, or play the feeling of them on a percussion instrument.
- Is it a loud feeling or a quiet one?
- Is it a soft feeling or a hard one?
- Does it make you feel good or bad?
- If the feeling was a place, what would it be (for example, a noisy town, a desert, a horrid smelly toilet)? Draw that picture.

✳ People who are like lovely music to be with

- Think about someone you really like being with.
- Paint the energy of this person.
- Is it a calm or gentle energy, or perhaps one full of life?
- How would you describe it?
- Play on the percussion instruments what you feel like when you are with this person.
- Show it in movement.

✳ The worry bag

This exercise comes as direct inspiration from the story called *The Huge Bag of Worries*, by Virginia Ironside, which is an excellent children's therapeutic story.

- Willy's worries were all about the wobbly world he lived in. What are your worries?
- Make a worry bag and write all your worries on separate little notes then put them into your worry bag.
- Which are the ones you would like help with.
- Keep your worry bag safe. When one of your worries has ended, cross it out and put it in another bag you can make called 'PHEW!'

✳ Sitting by your worries

- Draw your worries and you.
- What are they doing to you? For example, do you feel like you are being attacked by your worries, or drowning in them, or getting lost inside them?
- Now imagine you are sitting by the side of your worries. Or imagine you are flying high above your worries with a view of the whole of your life below, of which your worries are only a very small part. Or think of flowing with your worries, like a boat on a river. Trees that bend in the wind do not break.
- Draw the one of these images which you like best. Draw your worries in the picture.

For an anxious child, it can really help to actively imagine himself having a different relationship with his worries, or to make them smaller.

The following exercises are for children like Joe

✻ The giggle pool

This exercise aims to help a child like Joe to get back into the world of sensation, and to explore, as a toddler would, water, sand, clay and so on (whatever you have available). But for some children like Joe the invitation to make a mess may be refused, as it will be seen as too threatening. If so, downgrade the exercise – for example, to just drawing a Giggle Pool, or making one with Play-Doh® or plasticine.

> Make a Giggle Pool for yourself in the sand-pit, but your own version of a super fun place like that. Here are some water/ping-pong balls/marshmallows/balloons/clay/finger-paints/soil/bubbles/plasticine/leaves. Use whatever you like.

✻ Floppy jelly on the cushions

This exercise aims to help a child like Joe to get back to the world of his body, the world of physical sensation, instead of living in the world of his head. It is also about practising letting go, but into something safe and soft such as a pile of cushions. If, again, the cushions are too threatening, try to downgrade the exercise, and play something else physical instead, like rolling on big beach balls; a pillow fight; or running towards each other, each holding a cushion, so that you crash into each other. If you are playing 'floppy jelly', you will need to model it first as fun and safe, as children like Joe can easily feel silly, embarrassed or exposed. Such children also need adult models for letting go because many of them have not had any. So avoid getting the child to do something and you just watching. This exercise is very much a shared experience, a 'doing it together'.

Finally, children like Joe tend to need to get up quickly in order to re-establish control, so encourage them to languish on the cushions, to drift.

> Here is a big pile of cushions. We could fall on them or roll on them, or we could have a pillow fight.
> Or let's play floppy jellies. We both fall down like floppy jellies that have got so flopped they have finally flopped over.

☼ Do you ever feel like a straight line?

Do you ever feel rather like a straight line as Joe did?
If you ever feel like one of the pictures, or that life is like that, colour it in.

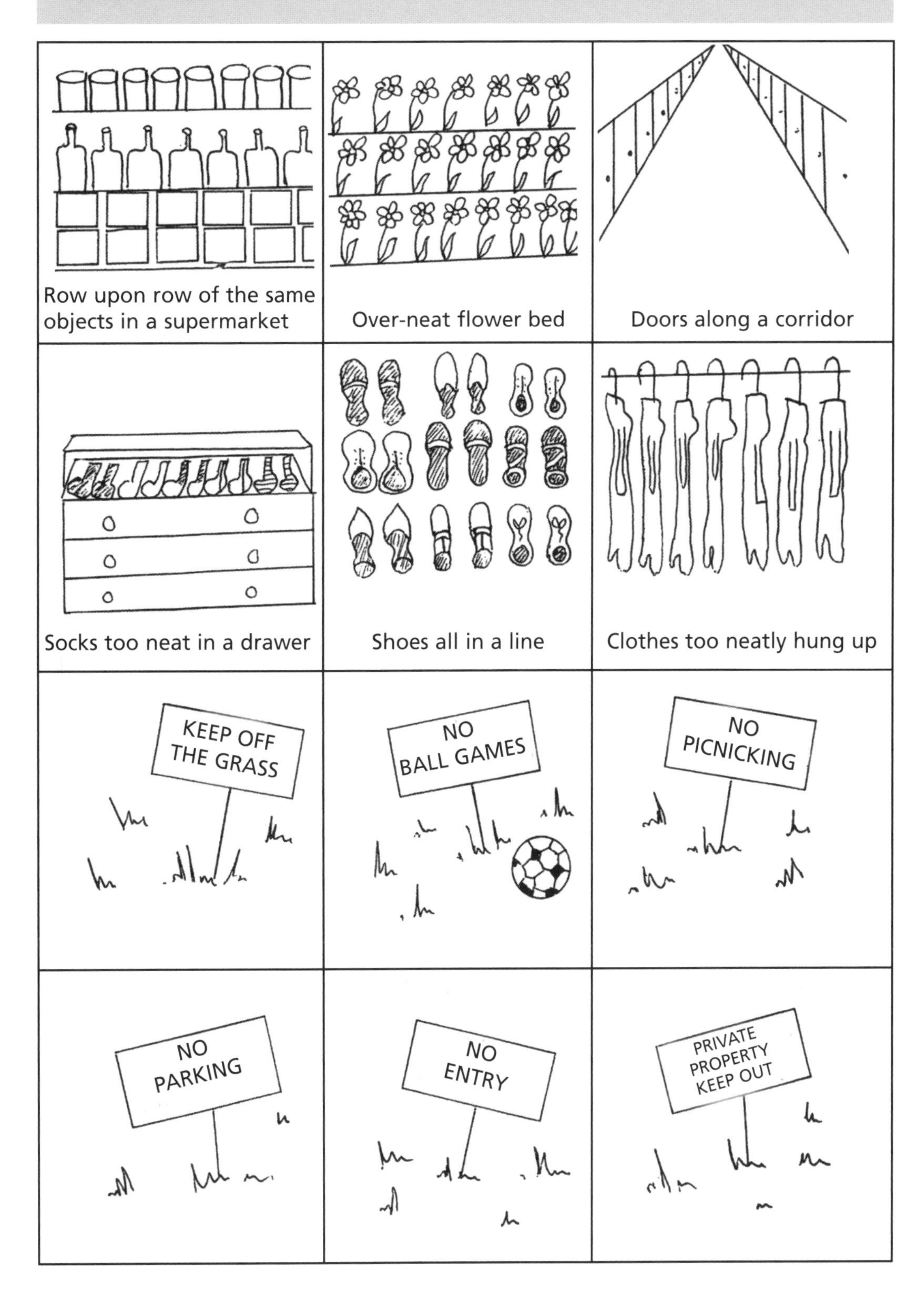

Figure 10
Straight lines

✳ Zabadabadoo!!!!! feelings

This exercise is designed for a child like Joe to try out more expansive, freer ways of being, and to enter into the creative realm of imagination and humour via a route of funny, amazing or absurd imagery. If you wait for a child who has cut himself off from play and fun to reconnect with them of his own accord, without inviting him back into their delights, you could be waiting for a long, long time. But, again, tailor this next exercise to minimise his embarrassment and maximise his fun.

Draw the feeling of, make or play out a sound for, or do a movement for:

- A waterfall
- A fairground slide
- A big belch
- Standing in a cow pat
- An apple dropping off the tree
- A singing sausage
- The Highland Fling
- Rolling down a grassy bank
- Being in a Giggle Pool
- A squelchy bog

✳ Yes we can

This is a super game for giving a child like Joe a real sense of what it is like to have fun, to be exuberant, free and imaginative with another person. The adult equivalent is that moment when two or more people are totally inspired and exhilarated over some creative endeavour or idea. Visits into the absurd can offer a very effective transportation for children who have got stuck in a way of being that is far too serious.

In this game you say something to end the sentence, 'Yes we can . . . '. Say the first thing that comes into your mind.
You might say 'Yes we can eat five hundred bananas in one minute', or 'Yes we can zip to the moon for a picnic'. And then whatever you say, we will both mime it in whatever way we like.
And then it's my turn, I will say 'Yes we can . . . ' and then again we both do it, and then it's your turn again and then it's my turn again.

Spend only about 30 seconds doing each of your and the child's 'yes we can' activities. This is to keep the momentum and minimise any embarrassment.

✳ 'Let's . . . ' in half a minute flat

This exercise is about inviting the over-serious child into the delightful world of shared creative activity. You can do any of the things listed below (either in reality, or by mime in imagination). The point is to do this exercise very fast – allowing just half a minute for each activity. This is so that it does not allow the child's spoiling or serious mind voices to come out and say to him, 'Don't'; 'Don't, it's too messy'; 'Don't, it's too silly'; or 'Don't, because if you do something awful will happen.'

- Let's make a mudpie with soil or sand or mud or clay.
- Let's make a mess on this piece of paper with clay, or soil or moistened cake-mix. Let's get our fingers to sink into its sogginess and squeeze it and paddle it about.
- Let's do a finger-painting.
- Let's start a drawing, but with no idea of what we will draw.
- Let's draw with our feet, not our hands (you need to take your socks off for this and hold the pencil in-between your toes).
- Let's play torpedoing boats in the sink, and make the boats out of paper.
- Let's blow some bubbles.
- Let's eat a very gooey, sticky meal together with our fingers.
- What else shall we do a 'Let's' with?

✳ People energies

This is for heightening the child's awareness of the energetic states of the people in his life. He may, for example, have unconsciously modelled his own energy on that of his depressed mother or his anxious father. The exercise is also for him to experiment with and rehearse different ways of being energetically. For example, he may really enjoy doing loud crashing on the cymbal, and so rehearse a more confident and assertive way of being. To help him sustain a new energy, you may want to play an instrument alongside him. Again, for a child like Joe, this may be one of the very few times that he has experienced the exhilaration of shared energetic exuberance. He may really get a taste for it. *But be careful not to upstage him in your playing*. Rather, just amplify what he is doing. To explain the concept of emotional energy to a child, you may have to demonstrate it.

- Show the different energies of the most important people in your life.
- Take each one in turn and:

  Move their energy

  Play it out in music

  Draw it
- How do you think their energy has affected your energy?
  Now play your own energy, the one you feel a lot of the time.
  What are the good things about being like this?
  What are the not good things?
- Play on the instruments how you would like your energy to be.

Tessa, who said she was bored a lot of the time, drew her mother's energy as a chewed piece of string, her father's energy as a still lake and her own as a pot of lard.

✳ Letting go and hanging on

Many children (and adults) when they say they want to 'really let go' mean that they want to 'let go while still holding on'. This is because, as we have seen, letting go is sometimes linked in the minds of children like Joe with something awful happening. So this exercise is for making children be more aware of both these pulls.

- Draw what you would do if you were as free as a bird, if you could do anything you like, and not be told off for it.
- What would you do?
- What do you imagine it would feel like?
- How might it feel great?
- How might it feel scary?
- Now draw you when you don't let go, but instead do everything the way it should be done.
- Draw what it feels like when you feel dull.
- Draw you when you feel too much like Joe.

✳ 'I'll be the strict person and you be the stroppy child'

This exercise is a good one for too-good children.

I will be a strict adult, and everything I ask you to do, you say 'Don't want to' or 'No' or 'Can't'.

What does it feel like to say 'No' instead of 'Yes' to an adult who wants something from you, or who wants you to do something?

What can happen if children like Joe suddenly discover and start to live their previously squashed life-force?

When 'undrawn' children like Joe do discover their life-force, be aware that it may come out angrily or rebelliously or destructively before it comes out constructively. Sometimes it may appear as an immediate burst into life and creativity, at others it can be the opposite: a burst into rage, or anger spinning out of control.

How to listen to children who are wobbly from a trauma

Listen to the child without inferring what he 'must be' feeling: for example, 'You must be furious with Daddy for leaving you.' The child may not be feeling that at all! You need to listen clearly, without putting on to the child what *you* would feel if it happened to you. It can be difficult for people not to assume that the child's psychology is the same as theirs.

You need to be able to stay with the child's feelings, however painful, without getting into advice-giving, into 'Look, what you need to *do* is . . . ', which neatly moves the child away from his feelings into thinking about action. (This can make you feel better, but blocks the child's feelings.) You also need to listen without cross-examining, or asking question after question.

Show the child through empathic response that you have really understood his perception of the event; do not tell him, or imply, how he should be seeing it. He may well tell you this through a drawing, or enacting a story, so it is good to reply and offer your empathy through story and through *metaphorical* accuracy, rather than directly.

A person can *talk* about feelings for hours on end without ever feeling them. This will not release that person from the trauma's effects. So, as the listener, you need to be with the child in a very open, empathic, unscared way, so that the child eventually feels safe enough to withstand the full intensity of his feelings, for example, while he howls and howls, or while he shakes or screams out the fear he has felt.

CONSIDERING FURTHER COUNSELLING OR THERAPY FOR CHILDREN WHO ARE ANXIOUS OR WHO CANNOT LET GO

Counselling for the child like Willy

The counsellor or therapist can help the child sort out his feelings of inner chaos or confusion. She can help him understand what caused such a tangle in the first place. If a wobbly child has access to a counsellor or therapist, who has a real sense of inner calm, rather than a pseudo-calm covering agitation, he can gradually integrate this experience and develop a self-soothing function. This means being able to soothe his own states of stress and tension, quieten himself down, or knowing when he needs to find someone who will help calm him and going to that person.

If someone helps an anxious child to process and think about feelings that feel too much, too muddled or too overwhelming, he can experience immense relief. With an empathic other, a child can feel connected to his emotional experience rather than simply flooded by it.

As we have said, a wobbly child is a child who is too full of difficult feelings that he has not been able to process and digest properly. To be able to digest them, he needs someone to help him. It is the children who never got this help at home or at school who in adulthood may turn to drugs, alcohol or smoking to calm themselves. When a child is persistently plagued by wobbly, anxious feelings, therapy or counselling can offer a safe place from which he can look at the intense feelings that always underlie anxiety.

It feels very safe to be with someone who really understands about painful feelings, and who can keep thinking on your behalf, when you feel lost in or overwhelmed by the maze of your own feelings; someone who can withstand the intensity of your chaos and wobbliness when you feel that maybe you cannot. Such help can enable the child to build a stronger self. An example of this comes from Winnicott (a psychoanalyst) who said of one of his child therapy clients: 'Gabrielle showed growing confidence now in my ability to tolerate muddle, dirt . . . incontinence and madness' (Winnicott, 1980, p105) – meaning that, as a result, the child could now manage them better herself.

If a child is wobbly from post-traumatic stress, counselling or therapy is essential. To process and work through major trauma in a child's life so that it does not keep haunting him, very particular attention is required. Hence the need, usually, for a very skilled counsellor or psychotherapist.

Counselling for the child like Joe

Sometimes, without therapy, the internalised oppressor – the 'shoulds' and 'mustn'ts' in the child's mind – continue to rule. He obeys them unthinkingly. They have gained too much of a stranglehold and why would they not, with no challenge? As the Jesuits say, 'Give us a child from nought to five, and we've got him for life.' And if a child sits on the fire of his passionate feelings for too long, the fire can go out.

Early conditioning, or habitual behaviour linked to compliance, to defending against strong feelings, to being good all the time and not upsetting the apple-cart, can become part of the hard-wiring of the child's brain. These established ways of being can then be incredibly hard to break. Luckily, however, with powerfully good and expansive relational experiences, there can be change in terms of the forming of new neuronal connections in certain higher regions of the emotional brain. The therapist can provide these experiences. (For more on this see Siegel, 1999; Schore, 1994).

> Psychotherapy takes place in the overlap of two areas of playing, that of the patient and that of the therapist. Psychotherapy has to do with two children playing together. The corollary of this is that where playing is not possible then the work done by the therapist is directed towards bringing the patient from a state of not being able to play into a state of being able to play. (Winnicott, 1971, pp38–52)

BIBLIOGRAPHY

Alvarez A, 1971, *The Savage God: A Study of Suicide*, Penguin, Harmondsworth.

Alvarez A, 1992, *Live Company*, Routledge, London.

Alvarez A, 1997, lecture given at 'Baby Brains' conference, Tavistock Clinic, London, July.

American Psychiatric Association, 1994, *Diagnostic and Statistical Manual of Mental Disorders: DSM-IV* 4th edn, American Psychiatric Association, Washington.

Andersen HC, 1994, *Hans Andersen's Fairy Tales* (Lewis N, trans), Puffin, Harmondsworth.

Auden WH & Kronenberger L, 1964, *The Faber Book of Aphorisms*, Faber & Faber, London.

Balint E, 1993, *Before I Was I: Psychoanalysis and the Imagination* (Mitchell J & Parsons M, eds), Free Association Books, London.

Balint M, 1955, 'Friendly Expanses – Horrid Empty Spaces', *International Journal of Psycho-Analysis* 36(4/5), pp225–41.

Bennett A, 1995, *The Madness of King George*, Faber & Faber, London.

Blume ES, 1990, *Secret Survivors: Uncovering Incest and its Aftereffects in Women*, John Wiley, Chichester/New York.

Bowlby J, 1973, *Attachment and Loss: Volume 2 – Separation, Anxiety and Anger*, Hogarth Press, London.

Bowlby J, 1988, *A Secure Base: Clinical Applications of Attachment Theory*, Routledge, London.

Carroll L, 1953, Letter of 21 May in *The Diaries of Lewis Carroll* (ed RL Green), Volume One, London.

Carroll L, 1994, *Alice's Adventures in Wonderland*, Puffin, Harmondsworth, (Originally published 1865).

Clarkson P, 1988, 'Ego State Dilemmas of Abused Children', *Transactional Analysis Journal* 18(2), pp85–93.

Clarkson P, 1989, *Gestalt Counselling in Action*, Sage, London.

Clarkson P, 1994, *The Achilles Syndrome: Overcoming the Secret Fear of Failure*, Element, Shaftesbury.

Cook D, 1991, *Second Best*, Faber & Faber, London.

Costello D, 1994, Personal communication.

Ehrenzweig A, 1971, *The Hidden Order of Art: A Study in the Psychology of the Artistic Imagination*, University of California Press, Berkeley/Los Angeles.

Fenichel O, 1990, *The Psychoanalytic Theory of Neurosis*, Routledge, London.

Freud S, 1917, 'General Theory of the Neuroses', in *Introductory Lectures on Psychoanalysis*, Vol 1 of *The Penguin Freud Library* (Richards A & Strachey J, eds, Strachey J, trans) (1973) Penguin, Harmondsworth.

Freud S, 1923 'Neurosis and Psychosis', pp209-18 in *On Psychopathology, Inhibitions, Symptoms and Anxiety*, Vol 10 of *The Penguin Freud Library* (Richards A & Strachey J, eds, Strachey J, trans), Penguin, Harmondsworth.

Freud S, 1926, 'Inhibitions, Symptoms and Anxiety', pp237–333 in *On Psychopathology, Inhibitions, Symptoms and Anxiety*, Vol 10 of *The Penguin Freud Library*, (Richards A & Strachey J, eds, Strachey J, trans), 1979, Penguin, Harmondsworth.

Glucksman M, 1987, 'Clutching at Straws: An Infant's Response to Lack of Maternal Containment', *British Journal of Psychotherapy*, 3(4), pp347–49.

Goldman D, 1993, *In One's Bones: The Clinical Genius of Winnicott*, Jason Aronson, Northvale, NJ.

Goleman D, 1996, *Emotional Intelligence*, Bloomsbury, London.

Hargreaves R, 1978, *Mr Worry,* World, Manchester.

Herman N, 1987, *Why Psychotherapy?*, Free Association Books, London.

Herman N, 1988, *My Kleinian Home: A Journey Through Four Psychotherapies*, Free Association Books, London.

Hopkins GM, 1985, *Poems and Prose*, (Gardner WH, ed), Penguin, Harmondsworth.

Johnson SM, 1994, *Character Styles*, Norton, New York.

Kahn MMR, 1991, *Between Therapist and Client: The New Relationship*, WH Freeman, New York.

Klein M, 1932, *The Psychoanalysis of Childhood*, Hogarth Press, London.

Kohut H, 1984, *How Does Analysis Cure?*, University of Chicago, London/Chicago.

Kohut H & Wolf ES, 1978 'The Disorders of the Self and Their Treatment', *International Journal of Psycho-Analysis*, 59, pp413–24.

Little M, 1990, *Psychotic Anxieties and Containment: A Personal Record of an Analysis with Winnicott*, Aronson, Northvale, NJ.

McDougall J, 1989, *Theatres of the Body: A Psychoanalytical Approach to Psychosomatic Illness*, Free Association Books, London.

MacLeod S, 1996, 'The Art of Starvation', Dunn, S, Morrison B & Roberts M (eds), *Mind Readings – Writers' Journeys Through Mental States*, Minerva, London.

Maslow AH, 1971, *The Farther Reaches of Human Nature*, Viking Penguin, New York.

Miller A, 1990, *Thou Shalt Not Be Aware: Society's Betrayal of the Child*, Pluto, London.

Milner M, 1987, *The Suppressed Madness of Sane Men*, Tavistock, London.

Nietzsche F, 1993, *The Sayings of Friedrich Nietzsche* (Martin S, ed) Duckworth, London.

Odier C, 1956, *Anxiety and Magical Thinking*, International Universities Press, New York.

Panksepp J, 1998, *Affective Neuroscience*, Oxford University Press, New York.

Phillips A, 1996, 'The Disorder of Uses; A Case History of Clutter', Dunn S, Morrison B & Roberts M (eds), *Mind Readings – Writers' Journeys Through Mental States*, Minerva, London.

Quiller-Couch A, 1979, *The Oxford Book of English Verse 1250–1918*, Oxford University Press, Oxford.

Rilke RM, 1939, *The Duino Elegies*, (Leishman JB & Spender S, trans), WW Norton, New York.

Rowan J, 1986, *Ordinary Ecstasy: Humanistic Psychology in Action*, Routledge & Kegan Paul, London.

Rycroft C, 1988, *Anxiety and Neurosis*, Maresfield, London.

Salinger JD, 1951, *The Catcher in the Rye*, Penguin, Harmondsworth.

Schore A, 1994, *Affect Regulation and the Origins of the Self – The Neurobiology of Emotional Development*, Lawrence Erlbaum Associates, New Jersey.

Segal J, 1985, *Phantasy in Everyday Life: A Psychoanalytical Approach to Understanding Ourselves*, Penguin, Harmondsworth.

Shah I, 1966, *The Exploits of the Incomparable Mulla Nasrudin*, Picador, London.

Siegel DJ, 1999, *The Developing Mind*, The Guildford Press, New York.

Stern DN, 1985, *The Interpersonal World of the Infant*, Basic Books, New York.

Sunderland M, 1993, *Draw On Your Emotions*, Speechmark Publishing, Bicester.

Sunderland M, 2000, *Using Story Telling as a Therapeutic Tool with Children*, Speechmark Publishing, Bicester.

Thomas D, 1995, 'Under Milk Wood' in *The Dylan Thomas Omnibus*, Phoenix, London.

White A, 1979, *Beyond The Glass*, Virago, London.

Wickes FG, 1988, *The Inner World of Childhood: A Study in Analytical Psychology*, 3rd edn, Sigo Press, Boston, MA.

Williams G, 1997, *Internal Landscapes and Foreign Bodies*, Tavistock, London.

Winnicott DW, 1960, *The Family and Individual Development*, Tavistock, London.

Winnicott DW, 1971, 'Playing: A Theoretical Statement', in *Playing and Reality*, Tavistock, London.

Winnicott DW, 1980, *The Piggle: An Account of the Psychoanalytic Treatment of a Little Girl*, Penguin, Harmondsworth.

Helping Children with Feelings

Margot Sunderland, illustrated by Nicky Armstrong

This is a ground-breaking pack of nine beautifully illustrated stories which have been designed to help children who are troubled in their lives. The stories act as vehicles to help children think about and connect with their feelings. Each is accompanied by a guidebook that will prove a vital resource when using the stories. Featured below are details about five of the titles and an accompanying handbook.

Using Story Telling as a Therapeutic Tool with Children

This practical manual begins with the philosophy and psychology underpinning the therapeutic value of story telling. It shows how to use story telling as a therapeutic tool with children and how to make an effective response when a child tells a story to you. It is an essential accompaniment to the series: Helping Children with Feelings. Covers such issues as:

- Why story telling is such a good way of helping children with their feelings;
- What resources you may need in a story-telling session;
- How to construct your own therapeutic story for a child;
- What to do when children tell stories to you;
- Things to do and things to say when working with a child's story.

108pp, illustrated, paperback
Order code: 002-4720

Willy and the Wobbly House

Helping children who are anxious or obsessional

Willy is an anxious boy who experiences the world as a very unsafe wobbly place where anything awful might happen at any time. Joe, the boy next door, is too ordered and tidy to be able to ever really enjoy life. Willy longs for order while Joe longs for things to wobble. However, when they meet Mrs Flop she tells them they don't have to put up with feeling as they do. At her suggestion they visit the Puddle People who help them break out of their fixed patterns and find far richer ways of living in the world.

Storybook: 32pp, A4, full colour throughout, wire-stitched
Guidebook: 60pp, A4, illustrated, wire-o-bound
Order code: 002-4774

The Frog Who Longed for the Moon to Smile

Helping children who yearn for someone they love

Frog is very much in love with the moon because the moon once smiled at him. Now he spends all his time gazing at the moon and dreaming about her. He waits and waits for her to smile at him again. One day a wise and friendly crow helps Frog to see how he is wasting his life away. Eventually Frog takes the huge step of turning away from the moon. When he does, he feels a terrible emptiness and loneliness. He has not yet seen what is on the other side of him. When in time he looks around, he is lit up by everything he sees. All the time he has been facing the place of very little, he's had his back to the place of plenty.

Storybook: 32pp, A4, full colour throughout, wire-stitched
Guidebook: 48pp, A4, illustrated, wire-o-bound
Order code: 002-4776

A Nifflenoo Called Nevermind

Helping children who bottle up their feelings

Nevermind always carries on whatever happens! Each time something horrible happens to him he is very brave and simply says 'never mind'. He meets with all kinds of setbacks, bullying and disappointments but each time he just tucks his feelings away and carries on with life. However, he becomes so full of bottled-up feelings that after a time he gets stuck in a hedge. In addition, some of these feelings start to leak out of him in ways that hurt others. Luckily he happens upon a bogwert who helps him understand that his feelings do matter and should not be ignored. Nifflenoo then learns how to both express his feelings and stand up for himself.

Storybook: 36pp, A4, full colour throughout, wire-stitched
Guidebook: 48pp, A4, illustrated, wire-o-bound
Order code: 002-4775

A Pea Called Mildred

Helping children pursue their hopes and dreams

Mildred is a pea with dreams. She has great plans for her pea life. However, people are always telling her that her dreams are pointless as she is just another ordinary pea. As she is not prepared to be just another ordinary pea and let go of her dreams, she goes into a very lonely place. Eventually, with the help of a kind person along the way, Mildred ends up doing exactly what she has always dreamed of doing.

Storybook: 28pp, A4, full colour throughout, wire-stitched
Guidebook: 28pp, A4, illustrated, wire-o-bound
Order code: 002-4777

A Wibble Called Bipley (and a Few Honks)

Helping children who have hardened their hearts or become bullies

Bipley is a warm cuddly creature, but the trouble is someone has broken his heart. He feels so hurt that he decides it is just too painful to ever love again. When he meets some big tough Honks in the wood, they teach him how to harden his heart so that he doesn't have to feel hurt anymore. Bipley turns into a bully. To begin with he feels powerful but gradually he realises that the world has turned terribly grey. Luckily, Bipley meets some creatures who teach him how he can protect himself without hardening his heart.

Storybook: 44pp, A4, full colour throughout, wire-stitched
Guidebook: 60pp, A4, illustrated, wire-o-bound
Order code: 002-4778

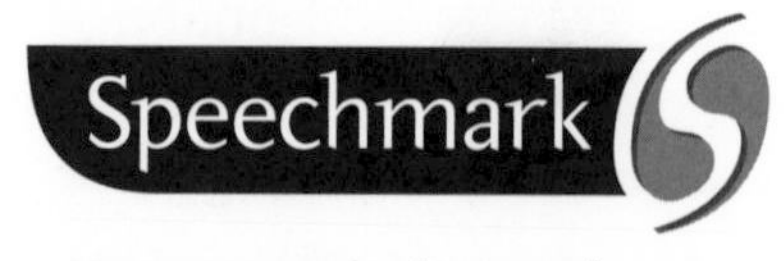

www.speechmark.net